AF342553

Breeding Food Animals

Live Food for Vivarium Animals

Breeding Food Animals
Live Food for Vivarium Animals

Ursula Friederich

and

Werner Volland

63 Black-and white photographs and drawings

KRIEGER PUBLISHING COMPANY

Malabar, Florida
2004

Original German Edition *Futtertierzucht: Lebendfutter für Vivarientiere* 1981
Original English Edition 2004

Printed and Published by
KRIEGER PUBLISHING COMPANY
KRIEGER DRIVE
MALABAR, FLORIDA 32950

Translated from the original German by Valerie Haeckey

Library of Congress Cataloging-in-Publication Data

Friederich, Ursula.
    [Futtertierzucht. English]
    Breeding food animals : live food for vivarium animals / Ursula Friederich and Werner
  Volland ; [translated from the original German by Valerie Haecky].
      p. cm.
    Includes bibliographical references (p.) and index
    ISBN 1-57524-045-9 (alk. paper)
     1. Live food. 2. Small animal culture. 3 Captive wild animals—Feeding and feeds.
  4. Vivariums. I. Volland, Werner. II. Title.

SF99.L58F7413   2004
636.08'55—dc22
                                          2003066105

     10 9 8 7 6 5 4 3 2

Contents

Foreword

Keeping animals requires that we take good care of them. This responsibility includes appropriate housing, the required amounts of heat, light, and humidity, as well as a natural varied diet that is rich in vitamins. This is pointed out in much of the literature on vivarium animals, and much good advice is given on how to go about it. But most of these feeding instructions are scattered throughout the literature and are difficult to find when needed. In addition, questions frequently arise as to how much of this advice is based on actual experience.

Two enthusiastic animal lovers and experienced keepers have now collected, reviewed, and tested all of these instructions: Ursula Friedrich, who has a diploma in biology, and Werner Volland, who is an animal caretaker. Their list of food animals extends from the smallest fruit flies to the larger rodents. The reader will find clear and well-structured instructions, including mostly unknown tricks, and information on the advantages and disadvantages of the various breeding setups. The reader can be assured that following these instructions will result in the successful breeding of food animals.

Thanks to this book, the keeper who conscientiously considers the well-being of his or her animals can feed a varied diet even when the by rights recommended diet of "meadow plankton" is not available. It is no longer necessary to fall back onto an inadequate and monotonous diet of mealworms.

I would like to express special thanks for this book to the authors and the publisher. One has to wonder, why such an urgently needed book on recurring feeding issues has not been published sooner in the community of vivarium enthusiasts.

Heinz Wermuth

Preface

The number of people who in their spare time enjoy unusual pets like amphibians and reptiles, rare birds, small mammals, fish, predatory insects and invertebrates, grows every year. Many of these animals have one thing in common: in the long term they require live food to stay healthy and strong, or even breed.

While there were plenty of untouched natural places and the use of insecticides was mostly unknown, vivarium enthusiasts had an easy time from spring to fall. Insects and other small animals could easily be found in meadows, in bushes, and in ponds. But even then husbandry was not without its challenges, as the appropriate food was often not available in winter, and breeding food animals was either unknown or too complicated.

Today it is getting harder and harder to catch enough live food, even in summer. In addition, many vivarium enthusiasts live in cities; they might at best have time to go hunting for food on the weekend. This is why the breeding of food animals is becoming more and more relevant. With this book we want to prove that this is not too difficult, even for the vivarium hobbyist. The book describes the fundamentals of breeding food animals. The specific instructions include all the necessary details and many practical tips from our own experiences with our breeding setups or from the experiences of other vivarium enthusiasts. This book covers only setups that can be kept throughout the year in the house, on a balcony, or in the yard, and that demand only a reasonable amount of time, effort, and investment. We also refrained from including breeding instructions for animals that could easily get into the food in your pantry or that would otherwise be difficult to control, such as the Mediterranean flour moth, the Indian meal moth, bacon beetles, red flour beetles, and a variety of cockroaches.

We are aware that we cannot get into all the details, and that some lesser known food animals are not included; otherwise, the book would have been twice as thick. Most importantly we want to show vivarium enthusiasts the possibilities, how they can start their own food animal culture with simple tools and at a low cost. In time, they will find their own preferred methods that meet their own special requirements. In addition we show how by using technology in a reasonable way and by devising well thought out work procedures it is possible to maintain large-scale food animal setups. We hope that this "recipe book" inspires you to more variety in the menus of your vivarium animals, which is essential for the successful keeping and well-being of the animals.

Dr. Heinz Wermuth, former main curator at the Staatliche Museum für Naturkunde in Stuttgart, then called Ludwigsburg, did not just encourage the writing of this book, but also critically reviewed the manuscript for the first edition; our heartfelt thanks go to him.

Support from our publisher Eugen Ulmer, especially from the editors Mr. Ulrich Commerell and Mr. Michael Kokoscha, and our open cooperation over the years, have created a lasting relationship.

Many people have over the years contributed to the creation and improvement of this book. We give them all our heartfelt thanks! We can only name a few: Mr. Hans Schneider, Reutlingen, reviewed the chapters on feeding fish. Prof. Dr. Werner Frank, Stuttgart-Hohenheim, provided us with valuable information on parasites in food animals. And Mr. Karl Friedrich Hohenstein, lawyer in Stuttgart, advised us in legal matters. The Wilhelma Zoological-botanical garden in Stuttgart supported us in many ways. Mrs. Renate Dieter, Stuttgart, typed the final manuscript of the first edition. Mrs. Maria Röthlin, Lucerne, wrote the first reader letter to U.F. Her hints, questions, and suggestions led to a lively exchange of thoughts. We share our joy about the publication of this third edition with all those who contributed to it with their knowledge.

Stuttgart and Lauchheim-Röttingen in February of 1997

Ursula Friedrich
Werner Volland

Introduction

We carry considerable responsibility for the vivarium animals we keep. Before concentrating on one special topic, their diet, we must make sure that all the other husbandry requirements of our animals are met; that is, sufficient room to move around, correct temperature and humidity, and a species-appropriate enclosure. The diet of vivarium animals poses big problems for many keepers since many of them require a diet supplemented by live food, and sometimes a diet that consists completely of live food. There are three ways in which to solve this problem: live food is caught outdoors, it is bought at a pet store or from a breeder, or we breed it ourselves. This book is about the third option and it provides the necessary information on it. Again and again, we read that insects netted in meadows and other wild caught foods are the best that we can offer our vivarium animals. This, however, is not true without reservations! Consider the harmful substances to which wild animals are exposed in many areas. Of course, wild-caught food has one distinct advantage: it is more varied. However, three days of rain can be detrimental to netting live insects in a meadow. Besides, this kind of food is only available for a few months of the year. Breeding your own food animals makes you independent of such vagaries. Knowing how young animals suffer if there is not enough food available, anyone who tries to raise 50 juvenile frogs or 30 chameleons without their own breeding setup should rightfully be called "irresponsible."

Of course, many objections can be made to the assertion that "captive-bred food animals are best." The biggest difference in wild food is that *we* determine the quality. Many vivarium enthusiasts have proven for years with their successes in husbandry and breeding that optimally fed and bred food animals are at least equal, if not superior, to wild-caught ones.

However, each food animal can only be as valuable as the food on which it is fed. This is the guiding principle for every food animal breeding setup; it will be our companion throughout this book.

Live Food for Vivarium Animals

Basic Considerations

The Significance of Live Food

"Eating and being eaten" is often quoted after someone has seen a documentary on television that shows how a lion kills a zebra, a crocodile drowns a bird, or a praying mantis grasps a grasshopper and starts eating it. In fact, about one third of all animals feed exclusively or partially on other animals, most of them taking live prey. A large number of vivarium animals fall into this group. To better understand their needs, one should think about what role food, and especially live food, plays in their daily rhythm and their whole life.

All animals must eat organic materials—that is, other living beings—in order to absorb the elements that they need for their metabolism: proteins, carbohydrates, fats, water, minerals (salts), and vitamins. The need for water and minerals is usually only partially satisfied by food. Live food has the advantage that it contains all these substances in the freshest state .The contents of the digestive system of the prey animals are also important; they usually feed on plants or other animals that are not on the predator's menu, which indirectly enriches the predator's diet. When they consume live foods, predators also ingest indigestible components, such as chitin shells and insect wings—roughage that activates the digestive system. In addition, animals that eat a varied diet are more common than those that specialize in certain foods, so that a monotonous diet is rarely the rule. This should encourage keepers to take advantage of the large palette of live food animals that are available.

In the wild, food is rarely abundant enough to allow animals to be picky; rather, they must eat at any available opportunity. They must also pay attention to their own survival, as most predators can easily become prey themselves. In captivity, the threat of being eaten is usually missing and the cage world offers few excitements. The stimulation offered by live food is psychologically important.

Larger animals survive periods of fasting without damage. Often such fluctuations are part of the natural rhythm of plenty and lack. However, young animals require regular feedings; therefore, they spend more time looking for food. Different groups and species of animals use differing strategies to acquire their prey. Some sit in waiting, as for example, predatory grasshoppers as well as the alligator snapping turtle and the Mata Mata turtle. Many pursue their prey. Of those, some are constantly looking for food, as for example fish, while others look for food at certain times only, like bats, lizards, and snakes. Climate, breeding seasons, and pregnancy influence feeding behaviors throughout the year.

Fortunately, many vivarium animals adapt easily and accept dietary substitutes. A case in point is all the dry and flake foods that are available to the aquarium enthusiast. It is not our intent to criticize the use of commercial foods or to diminish the value of homemade prepared food mixtures, such as gelatin cubes. Many fish, frogs, turtles, and lizards can be well fed using them. However, for most animals, successful breeding requires feeding with live foods, and there are plenty of untrainable vivarium animals that only accept live or recently killed food.

Catching, Buying, Breeding

Catching, buying, or breeding one's own are the three most common ways in which to acquire live food. Usually, the vivarium enthusiast will make use of all three options and combine them to match his or her needs. Depending on the time of year, number of animals kept, spare time available, space and financial resources, one or the other option may be preferred. How to catch live food animals has been described extensively in other books, so it is not discussed further here.

Pet stores rarely offer more choices than mealworms, blowfly maggots, Tubifex worms, and brine shrimp. The number of specialized breeders has increased dramatically in recent times, so that almost all the food animals described in this book can also be bought. This is also important since one requires breeding stock and other vivarium enthusiasts may not always be able to help. It is also possible that personal efforts do not yield enough food or that a breeding endeavor fails. Magazines for vivarium enthusiasts, reptile and amphibian societies, and the Internet can provide listings of suppliers.

Home-breeding food animals is the best way to guarantee a basic supply of live food for your vivarium animals. At the same time, it can be the starting point of a "food exchange ring," where vivarium enthusiasts coordinate the breeding and exchanging of live food animals, either on a regular basis or as needed.

This has the advantage that each person can specialize in one or two food animals and still be able to offer their animals a varied diet. However, such an undertaking requires that one live close to other vivarium enthusiasts who keep animals with similar requirements, and who are interested in collaboration.

Feeding Live Food to Vivarium Animals

It is extremely important that food animals be well fed. Harvest crickets and cockroaches whose bellies look full and larvae that are ready to molt. Insects that go through complete metamorphosis, like flies, should be fed for at least three, better five, days after they emerge from their cocoons. By this time, the females will have developed eggs and are nutritionally especially valuable. Other animals, like grindal worms, snails, and water fleas are harvested a few hours after they have been fed. When food animals are bought from pet stores or breeders, either for use as food or breeding stock, they are often starved because of either transportation or less-than-ideal husbandry. They should be fed before they are offered as food.

Food animals, especially insects, are very suitable as carriers for vitamins and mineral powders. Before using these insects as food, they can be put into a bag and shaken with a small amount of powder. This is also a good way of feeding calcium and vitamin D_3 supplements. Several brands formulated for vivarium animals are available.

All efforts to offer well-fed food animals are of no use, if the animals are not hungry and the food remains in the cage uneaten for hours or days. Therefore, it is best to wait until the animals are truly hungry before feeding them. At their natural feeding times, they will most probably attack and devour the offered food immediately. Ideally, the animals should be able to eat the offered food within a short time, and they should be observed while they eat. The advantages are obvious: You can make sure that all your animals are eating and that they appear healthy and strong. Food can be offered individually to weaker and smaller animals and those that are always hungry can be restrained. The water in the vivarium remains unpolluted, the vivarium furniture unchewed, and the vivarium animals attentive and lively.

However, even supervised feedings do not always go smoothly. Many animals, especially newly acquired ones, are so shy that they will only eat when undisturbed. To keep from disturbing them, the food can be placed into their enclosure shortly before they become active and possibly interested in eating.

Many vivarium enthusiasts have day jobs; this often leaves them with little time to observe their animals for longer periods. In this case, weekends can be used to catch up for time lost during the week. Controlled feeding does not mean that food should be offered by hand and all the animals have to do is grab it. Searching for and chasing prey play a significant role in the lives of fish, birds, reptiles, amphibians, mammals and insects and require much time in the wild; these natural instincts should be preserved. After all, the goal is to have healthy, lively, and strong animals. Since in the wild food is not available regularly, portion-size should be varied: smaller prey more frequently at one time, and larger prey less often at another time, sometimes so much that the animals can stuff themselves, and sometimes only tidbits. Of course, this will vary from species to species. A monitor lizard can fast for up to three weeks, while baby fish would barely survive one day of fasting.

The size of the prey is to be such that it can be overpowered, sometimes only barely. If there are doubts, the animals should be observed to allow intervention if necessary. Uneaten prey can be dangerous, especially to young animals, when the prey becomes the predator. I remember a *Cyclops* attacking juvenile fish, and the case of a small day gecko that was mortally wounded by a grasshopper or maybe a spider. If food animals can find food in the vivarium, this risk is reduced. Nocturnal food animals pose a special threat for diurnal vivarium animals. It is important that, for example, crickets and mice have food available at night if they cannot be removed in the evening. It is better to take preventive measures than to end up sorry.

How are food animals offered? As often, there are several options. For the animals, it is most interesting and natural if they can find and subdue their own food. For this, a small number of food animals are placed into the aquarium or terrarium. If the vivarium is large and heavily planted, the food animals will quickly find shelter and become unreachable. In this case, and for birds and mammals, it is recommended to feed from a bowl or by hand using tweezers, pincers, or a needle.

The bowl should be made of a smooth, opaque material with sides that are high enough to prevent mealworms or other larvae from escaping. Glass dishes are only suitable if they are buried in the substrate, as vivarium animals will often bump into the sides, not understanding that they can see their prey but cannot get at it. Use a bowl with a sufficiently large diameter and plant it firmly. Since this method is primarily used by vivarium enthusiasts who are at work during the day, and the bowl is placed in the vivarium in the morning; also provide something to eat for the food animals.

Animals that have settled in can be taught to accept food from tweezers, pincers, a needle, or directly from the hand. Please, do the latter only if there is no potential for serious bites!

Tweezers should be made of wood, plastic, or metal and their tips must be rounded. Do not let the animals bite on them because they can injure their jaws. Grasp insects by their wings or at least two legs; hold grasshoppers and crickets by their rear-most legs, otherwise, they can escape easily. To be less conspicuous, prey can be offered to shy animals on the tip of a piece of wire—not skewered! A long piece of steel wire with a diameter similar to a paper clip (Schulte, 1980) or the ends of an electric wire with the copper wire bared can be used as needles. To make a feeding needle, a 10-centimeter-long piece of wire is attached to a stick. The total length and diameter of the needle and wire depend on the size of the food animal used. When the animal grabs the prey, the needle or wire must be withdrawn carefully.

You can find additional information in the sections on specific food animals. If you have more specific questions on feeding your vivarium animals, refer to care information on the species in question.

Food Animals and Conservation

Even though the topic of this book is the breeding of food animals, it is necessary to mention regulations. A number of amphibians and reptiles are protected federally, statewide, or locally, or there are limits to their taking or breeding. If you need lizards or amphibians to feed your vivarium animals, make sure you know the regulations for your state. In general, we do not encourage the keeping of animals that feed exclusively on amphibians or reptiles and that do not accept substitutes. It will always be problematic to obtain food items for them, and you must consider whether you are comfortable using animals as food items that you would also keep as pets.

A number of insects are also protected, and some of them, for example stick insects, are illegal to keep and breed in several states. Some food animals can only be acquired, kept, bred, or shipped with a permit. Before collecting or breeding food animals, make sure you are familiar with the regulations for the area where you live.

Breeding Food Animals

Resaon for Breeding

At first glance it seems unnecessary to breed food animals at home. Pet stores and breeders conveniently provide all sorts of live foods that can be supplemented by catching additional food animals in meadows and ponds. In practice, however, it is not quite this simple.

As mentioned earlier, wild-caught live food is an excellent option, if it comes from places that are not polluted by insecticides and other poisons; otherwise, the vivarium animals acquire illness or even death instead of a vitamin and mineral rich treat.

Few vivarium enthusiasts can simply walk out of the house to catch food animals; most will have to drive some distance. Then it becomes also a question of time and price whether it is economical to drive to the meadow or pond regularly. In addition, wild-caught food animals—the same as captive bred ones—should be fed to the vivarium animals as soon as possible as otherwise the nutritional value decreases. Wild-caught food is usually seasonal and often needs to be supplemented with captive-bred food animals anyway.

Commercially available food animals do not always meet quality standards and it is upsetting to spend the money and not receive food animals of the required quality. Another difficulty arises when the available portioning is impractical. What should you do with a pint of fruit flies if only two small frogs are hungry?

Even commercial breeders have delivery problems on occasion. In winter, shipping can be problematic because of the weather. How often has it happened, that an order of live crickets arrived frozen?

By breeding your own food animals, you become largely independent and with intelligent planning should have healthy, fresh live food available at all times. Since purchased live food must be stored in containers anyway, the step from keeping to breeding is small.

Most vivarium enthusiasts fear the additional work that arises with breeding. It would be wrong to say that houseflies and brine shrimp will proliferate on their own. Equally wrong would be to assume that breeding one's own food animals generates so much work that the vivarium enthusiast could not handle it. Appropriate containers and the right tools make the breeding process a lot easier. The necessary skills can be learned quickly, and after a time everyone becomes adept enough that it works out smoothly. Finally, you wonder why you hesitated so long before breeding your own food animals.

Of course, any vivarium enthusiast will ask whether it is worthwhile to keep one's own breeding setups for food animals. The answer to this question depends on many factors and it cannot be answered generally.

A hobbyist with much spare time might decide in favor of breeding even if he or she only keeps a few animals, and he or she might be more willing to invest in a more labor-intensive breeding setup than someone who works long hours. The length of each generation and the productivity rate of the setup are important criteria; for two water turtles, it is worth breeding earthworms, but breeding grasshoppers for two frogs is not worth the effort.

If you mistrust every food animal that you did not breed yourself, you will want to have as many different breeding setups as possible.

When planning breeding setups for food animals, domestic peace should also be considered. It is rare indeed that the whole family is enthusiastic about animals. Other family members do not always share our enthusiasm. Since in most cases there is no completely separate area available to set up the breeding containers, a good amount of goodwill and tolerance from partners, parents, or children is required. In addition, not everybody feels sympathetic towards earthworms or mice.

Breeding setups for food animals require space and cannot be completely hidden because of their size, noise, or smell. Even with the utmost care, flies will occasionally buzz around or grasshoppers will hop across the carpet. Food mixtures for the food animals must be prepared in the kitchen. Refrigerator and freezer space must be negotiated, and the sink and the bathtub are used for cleaning chores.

Let's make sure that our families and we ourselves are clear on this, so that we can enjoy our interesting and fascinating hobby for a long time without conflict!

Those who take a liking to breeding food animals and have enough space and business sense might consider expanding some of their breeding endeavors into a sideline or even mainline business. There should be no lack of customers for flawless food animals.

Time and Material Requirements

Taking care of breeding setups requires a certain amount of time, maybe ten minutes a day for each setup, 15-30 minutes for large setups. While feeding is taken care of quickly, cleaning and rearranging setups take more time. Breeding setups also need to be inspected for sufficient offspring and for mites and diseases that might require treatment. You might even enjoy watching cockroach courtship, the jumping of water fleas, or crickets eating their food!

Remember that only optimally nourished food animals can meet our requirements. They should breed well and provide vivarium animals with all necessary nutrients, including trace elements and minerals. Therefore, food animals should never be neglected and always be fed regularly. Depending on the species and population, this may be necessary daily or weekly. Feeding small amounts more often leads to better results than feeding than large amounts infrequently.

The basic setups vary greatly depending on the animals, and the available selection of containers is big enough that the initial cost to can be matched to any size wallet. With a little craftsmanship, many accessories can be homemade, which is of course cheaper than buying. More information on containers and equipment can be found in the descriptions for specific breeding setups. The container sizes are usually indicated as length x width x height...

Legal Aspects

One consideration before starting to breed food animals is whether you rent your home, your lease allows you to do this, and if you own your home, how it might affect your neighbors. Breeding grasshoppers is without problems in this regard. However, crickets will definitely create a disturbance with their chirping, mice bother with their strong smell, and escaped wax moths and their larvae can damage wallpaper, pictures, and furniture. Escaped cockroaches can spread so much in an old house that they cannot be controlled.

Apart from the legal side, it is important to consider other people when keeping any kind of animal.

Legal questions and problems that could arise from breeding food animals have been discussed little in the legal literature. A blanket prohibition against pets in an apartment or house lease is often not interpreted to prohibit the keeping of a small bird or one food animal breeding setup that does not disturb anyone. However, breeding insects commercially in an apartment most likely infringes the lease, since the apartment or house is usually rented exclusively for habitation. It can thus be assumed that breeding food animals is acceptable to feed one's own animals, as long as it does not exceed a reasonable size, does not damage the place, and does not bother the neighbors in any way.

When breeding some types of cockroaches, special care must be taken to prevent infestation of the apartment and beyond by escapees. We therefore strongly recommend against such breeding setups, as excellent substitutes are available. To a smaller extent a danger of infestation exists for the house cricket (*Acheta domesticus*), but it is easier to control.

If cockroaches or other pests have infested an apartment, the lease may require that the owner be informed, and the owner may terminate the lease on these grounds. In addition, the cost for extermination and other costs may have to be paid. In addition, if a neighboring apartment is infested with animals from a food animal breeding setup, this can create liability claims and obligations to pay for any damages.

This means that insects that escape from breeding setups, now designated pests, can lead to serious problems and one should be extremely cautious when keeping such "dangerous" animals.

This danger is less for animals whose breeding requires higher temperatures because they originate in warmer climates. However, this rule does not always hold true. Consider termites that were introduced into Hamburg, Germany, by ships; they adapted quickly to the cooler climate and caused considerable damage to wood structures.

Starting a Breeding Setup

The choice of food animals to breed depends primarily on the animals kept. In addition, personal considerations, like available time and space, dislike of certain food animals, and last but not least allergies, influence the decision. Some food animal species can trigger allergic sinus reactions or asthma in sensitive persons. This is a known risk for cockroaches, migratory locusts, mealworm beetles, mice, and rats. It also does not make sense to breed food animals that are easily acquired elsewhere, as for example water fleas if a pond is nearby, or mealworms if there is a nearby pet shop.

Ideally, as many vivarium animals as possible like the food animals that you breed, so that it is worth your effort. In this context, it is not completely out of place to consider food preferences when choosing vivarium animals!

If you wish to breed more than one kind of food animal, it is best to choose them such that they have very different nutritional properties. In that way, the vivarium animals have more diverse food choices. The following combinations come to mind: Water fleas + grindal worms (+ fruit flies); crickets + houseflies (+ wax moths); cockroaches + migratory locusts (+ crickets or mice).

How do you acquire the necessary breeding stock? First, you can ask other vivarium enthusiasts and ask for some breeding stock; otherwise, catch, trap, or collect in the wild. A large number of food animal species can also be bought from large-scale breeders.

How extensive does a breeding setup have to be to satisfy the needs of a person's vivarium animals? This question always arises at the beginning, but it is not easy to answer. The following procedure might help: Before acquiring any vivarium animals, an experienced keeper can be quizzed about their daily or weekly food requirements. There is little specific written information available on this as it depends much on the age, nutritional state, and possible pregnancy of the animal. Together with information on reproduction rates, which are mentioned for each food animal, it can be estimated how many food animals need to be "produced" for each animal per day or week. In order to increase the safety margin, a somewhat bigger starting point can be assumed. In case of excess food animals, they can be frozen or used to help out other vivarium enthusiasts. More often than we like, a breeding setup does not work as desired, either because of mistakes, or simply because animals are not machines that always work predictably. It is therefore safer and better to breed at least two kinds of food animals. All vivarium animals like variation, and it makes it easier to compensate for problems.

If vivarium animals are to reproduce, the required breeding setups must be created or expanded in due time. Since both the development times of the food animals as well as for the vivarium animals—from spawning, breeding, or egg laying to free swimming, birth, or hatching—are known, it is easy to make preparations. Unexpected offspring can be a problem, especially with live-bearing reptiles. Many a purchased male has given birth to a lively litter of young! In this case, it is a relief to have colleagues that can help out for the first few critical days until any ordered food animals arrive or the breeding setups are producing full-scale.

Even with much planning it is difficult to obtain and maintain a complete balance between the available food animals and the food needs of the vivarium animals. It helps to have a stable breeding environment, good instincts, and experience.

All the food animals described in this book, except for mice and rats, are exotherms. The sequence of generations depends therefore on the temperature at which the setups are kept: higher temperatures make for shorter development times than lower temperatures. Obviously, this can be exploited to control breeding volume. If the setup is kept at an intermediate temperature, raising or lowering the temperature can significantly influence the rate of reproduction.

This sensitivity to temperature can also be exploited when too many food animals are available, when a breeding setup is not needed for some time, or if you are not at home for an extended period. Quite a few food animals can be refrigerated without harm for a period of time. The animals can be cooled down quickly, within a day, but they should be warmed up to their optimal breeding temperature slowly, over 2-3 days. A small refrigerator with a 30-40 l (1-2 cf^3) capacity is well suited, does not take up much space, and prevents spousal displeasure; food animals are not unappetizing, but not everyone likes them next to their food.

Nutrition for Food Animals

We mentioned in the introduction that it is not irrelevant how the food animals are fed. The general motto should be: "Only the best is good enough!" In addition to specialized foods, high-quality regular foods fulfill this requirement: brewer's yeast, milk powder, wheat germ, soy flour, ready-to-use commercial baby foods, children's vitamin juices, and others.

It cannot be repeated often enough that all leaves, lettuces, fruits, and vegetables must be pesticide free. Especially insects, which provide the largest number of food animals, will die if they are fed greens that have been sprayed and have even traces of insecticides on them. Feeding grasshoppers with endive lettuce in winter leads to frequent bad surprises. If wild herbs are collected, those that grow at the edge of the road must be avoided; the bigger and busier the road, the further away from it picking should begin (220 yards for freeways, 110 yards for highways), because these plants contain large proportions of poisonous heavy metals. Care must be taken in vineyards and orchards to make sure the trees have not been sprayed recently. The safest method is to grow food plants in the backyard and to grow wheat germ for grasshoppers. It is usually safe to collect plants from fallow fields, meadows, and forests.

It is especially important to use fresh food that is free of mold and rotten parts as intestinal problems that can be fatal will often result from eating such foods. All suspicious parts should be cut or trimmed off. Thorough rinsing removes dirt, pests, and remaining traces of insecticides. In short, the food should be prepared as carefully as if it was for a family meal.

It is certainly general knowledge that vertebrates require sufficient amounts of calcium, phosphorus, and vitamin D for healthy skeletal and muscular development. Additional minerals (trace elements) and a number of vitamins are required for a healthy metabolism.

Food animals should therefore be fed a diet rich in vitamins and minerals. However, vitamins are easily destroyed by high temperatures, light, and oxygen from the air. Therefore, at least some vitamins should be made directly available to the vivarium animals. Too much as well as too little can be harmful: overdosing of vitamins causes similar symptoms as a lack of them. Since few data are available on how to dose vitamins for vivarium animals, they should be dosed carefully and the animals observed regularly.

Juveniles and pregnant females should also be fed supplements directly. For land animals, it is customary to dust the food animals with a calcium-mineral powder before feeding. Since insects (the primary subject of this book) run around and lose much of their powder quickly, make sure they are eaten promptly. For aquatic vivarium animals, the supplements can be dissolved in the water in which they live. Vitamins can be given in the same manner. Food animals should be able to eat easily. Yeast mixed with water is easily taken by water fleas and brine shrimp. Cut up fruits and vegetables that are placed in the container with the cut surface down on the substrate can be accessed better by for example the different species of beetles. For crickets, cockroaches and snails, food is placed with the cut surface facing up. For dried foods, it depends on their hardness whether they should be offered hole, in pieces, or even ground up. Different food animals also have varying preferences. Newly hatched crickets prefer finely ground food.

There are no precise studies available on the nutritional value of home-bred food animals. Only mealworms and wax worms have been studied more closely. Depending on their origin and thus probably their nutrition, varying results have been found for mealworms (Martin et al., 1976).

Hygiene and Breeding Setups

Just as the entry hall provides the first impression of person's home, the breeding setups say much about a vivarium enthusiast. Two things are significant for long-term success: Feeding the food animals regularly with highest-quality food items and painstaking cleanliness for the breeding containers and equipment.

The cause for nonproducing breeding setups usually can be traced back to lack of hygiene. Pests can get into the breeding setups and diseases are almost unavoidable. Feces and food leftovers offer a paradise for mites, bacteria, and if the humidity is elevated, for molds. Therefore, get into the habit of removing all food leftovers before offering fresh food. At regular intervals that depend on the size of the breeding group, the food animals should be moved to containers with fresh bedding. All equipment must be cleaned with hot water and dishwashing liquid as if they were your own dishes. They must be rinsed thoroughly with clean water afterwards. Do not use strong cleaners! If traces remain on the equipment or containers, sensitive animals like migratory locusts can be lost. It is recommended to have brushes and towels designated solely for cleaning breeding containers. Mouse and rat cages must be disinfected once a month so that they cannot spread diseases or parasites. Containers for insects, plankton, and water fleas must never be disinfected because these animals cannot tolerate even traces of disinfectants. It is best to simply brush aquariums for plankton and water fleas with clean water.

Breeding Setups

The size of a breeding setup depends on the size of the animals as well as the number of containers. Three glasses of *Drosophila* require about 0.04 m^2, while eight rat cages need 3 m^2! In addition, storage space for extra containers, tools, and food must be considered.

Assuming that an apartment has room for one to two midsized aquariums, vivariums, or cages, room for the food animal breeding containers can likely be found. With 0.5-1.0 m^2 there should be enough room even to breed food for animals that will only take live food.

What is the best location for a breeding setup? Many options also depend on the size of the breeding project and the layout of the living space. In an apartment, vivariums are usually kept on cabinets, shelves, racks or something similar. The

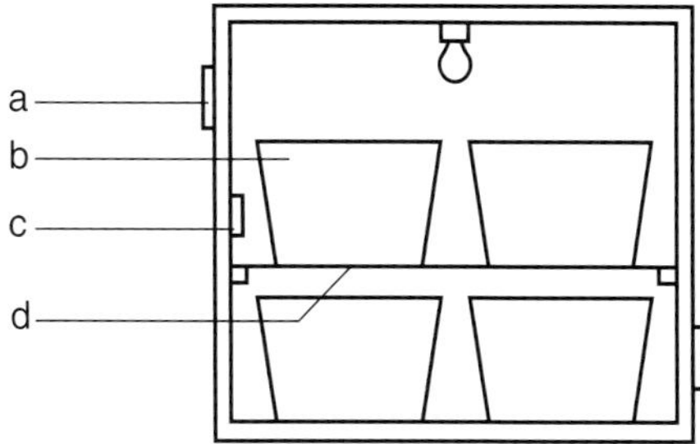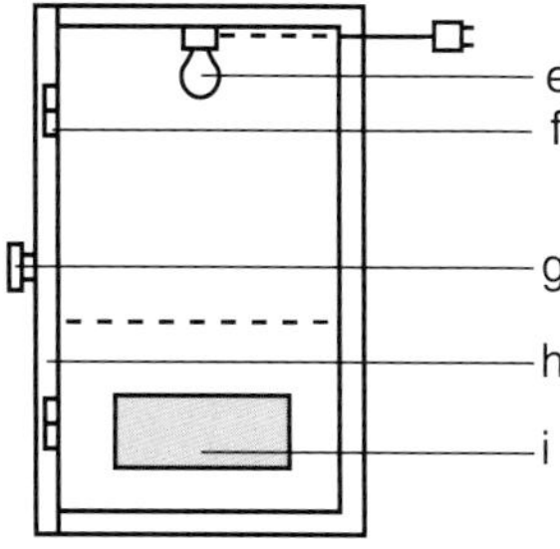

Fig. 1 Cabinet for breeding setups that tolerate dry air; front and side view. a) Ventilation top left, b) breeding container, c) magnetic lock, d) shelf (wire mesh), e) socket with ceramic heat emitter and connecting wire, f) door hinge, g) door handle, h) door, i) ventilation bottom right.

space underneath is used to store all sorts of accessories and could also be used for the food animal setups. A lamp ballast or even a warmed up pump can serve as a heat source. Just make sure that they still have enough airspace to prevent overheating. For breeding setups that can tolerate variations in temperature, as for example crickets or cockroaches, the heating from the central heating system or a woodstove during the cold period can be sufficient. Small, easily movable containers can be stored very high or in the bottom of a closet or shelf. For feeding and cleaning they can be carried to a more accessible location. Large containers that have built-in heating and/or lighting should be positioned in such a way that they can be serviced without contortions; otherwise, their care quickly becomes an unpleasant chore. Containers must never be placed where they are exposed to direct sunlight. They can overheat too quickly.

Since most breeding setups function best at temperatures between 25-30°C and heating containers individually requires a lot of electricity, it is more economic to store several containers together. Depending on the size of the breeding project, a chest or cabinet can be constructed. For food animals that require high humidity, the breeding containers need to be waterproof, or temperature- and humidity-controlled cabinets could be purchased, but this is expensive (Fig. 4) .

The following instructions are for building a dry cabinet (Figs. 1 & 2) that can be used for wax worms, crickets and the cockroach *Blaptica dubia*, and a climate-controlled cabinet (Fig. 3), for example for mealworms and death's-head cockroaches. The size of such a cabinet depends of course on the number and size of breeding containers. When calculating the volume, space for at least one extra container should be included.

Cabinet for Dry Breeding Setups: For the basic construction plywood or particleboard sheets that are 8-12 mm thick work well. Bottom, side panels, back panel, and cover can be glued and nailed together. Ventilation holes should be cut first into the side panels, as well as the drilled holes in a side panel or the cover for the electrical wires. For insulation the inside of the cabinet is lined with Styrofoam panels,

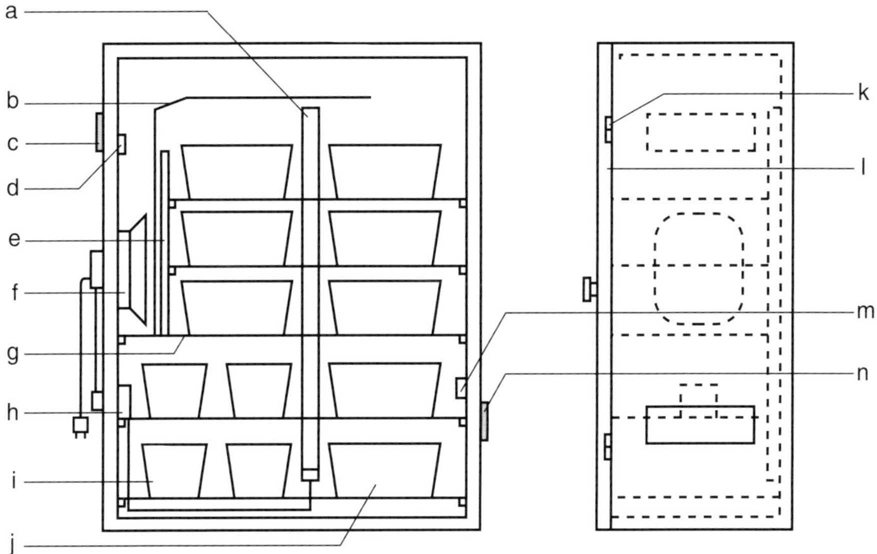

Fig. 2 Cabinet for breeding setups that tolerate dry air; front and side view. a) Fluorescent light, b) warm air disperser (metal heat conductor), c) ventilation top left, d) door lock, e) supports for shelves f) infrared heat emitter, g) shelf (wire mesh), h) light switch, i) breeding container, k) door hinge, l) door, m) thermostat, n) ventilation bottom right.

which have holes that match the ventilation holes. A good ceramic light socket that is rated to 150 watt is attached to the cover or side panel, or an infrared heat emitter can be used instead. The wood around the socket should be protected with a heat guard or a piece of heat-resistant insulating material that is wrapped into thick aluminum foil to protect it from overheating. This is not necessary if the cabinet is taller than 35 cm and the socket can hang in the center of the cabinet. This allows for a more even temperature, which can also be accomplished by mounting the socket on the side panel. For all setups that must be in the dark, an infrared heat emitter should be installed. Do not put any containers directly under this heat source, as they will get too hot. For additional safety, the heat

source can be covered with a metal sheet, which helps distribute the heat. An additional light socket for a work light can be installed. For breeding setups that need light, an incandescent bulb or a fluorescent light should be installed in addition to the infrared heat emitter (or the heat from the ballast can be used).

If necessary, a shelf similar to refrigerator wire-shelves can be added. The cabinet closes with a sliding or hinged door.

Temperature and Humidity-Controlled Cabinet: This cabinet is also constructed completely out of wood. Particle board that is 16 mm thick works well. A rectangular hole cut in each side panel will later be fitted with an adjustable ventilation cover. Holes for electrical wires should be drilled in the back panel. The side

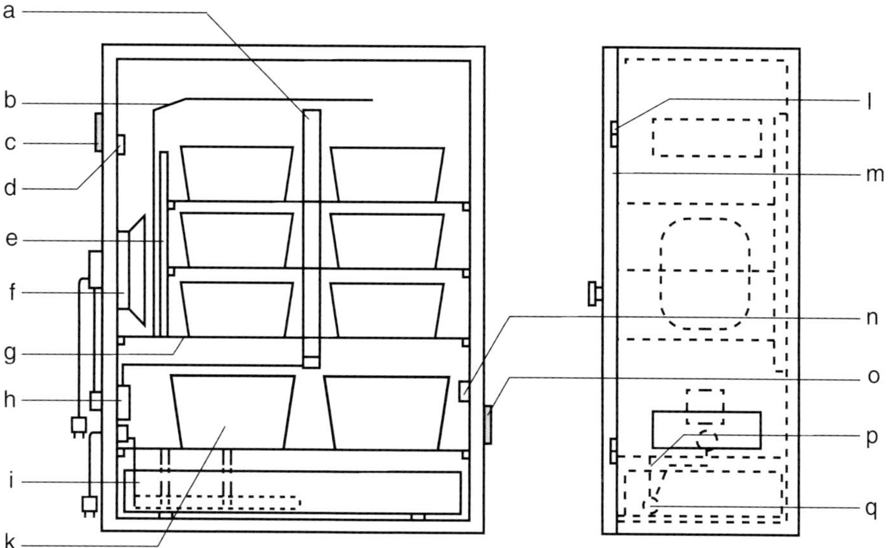

Fig. 3 Climatic chamber; front and back view. a) Fluorescent light, b) warm air disperser (metal sheet), c) top left ventilation hole, d) door lock, e) supports for shelves, f) heat emitter, g) shelf (wire mesh), h) light switch, i) water tray, k) breeding container, l) door hinge, m) door, n) thermostat, o) ventilation bottom right, p) mounting for heater, q) rheostat-controlled heater.

panels, floor, and cover panels are glued or screwed into a frame, the back panel attached and the door fitted with two to three hinges and an ordinary or magnetic lock. The inside of the cabinet must either be varnished or completely covered with aluminum foil to protect it against humidity. The side panels can be insulated with Styrofoam sheets.

A heat resistant tile or panel must be screwed or nailed to the middle of the side panel (see above) for the 100-150 watt infrared heat emitter and the wires threaded through.

At a distance of 10 cm from the heater, a sheet of aluminum that should be twice as long and wide as the heat emitter should be installed and be covered with heat resistant insulation material. The purpose of the aluminum panel is to disperse the heat so that the closest containers do not overheat.

If necessary, a fluorescent light and an incandescent work light can be installed. The sensor for the thermostat, which should definitely be added, goes in the middle of a side-panel.

To increase the air humidity, a shallow water tray should be set on the floor and the water heated with a 75-watt aquarium heater. A water temperature of 24-26°C can easily cause the air humidity to rise to 60-70% if the temperature in the cabinet is 24-25°C. If the air humidity does not reach the desired level, an aerator (bubbler) can be added to promote evaporation.

The heater must always be completely covered with water!
The breeding containers are arranged in several layers. Wood strips are nailed to the side panels at the desired height, then fitted with wire shelves similar to those used in refrigerators.
Temperature, humidity, and light can easily be controlled electronically. This opens many possibilities for vivarium enthusiasts that are also into electronic gadgetry.
If the cabinet is to be placed in the basement or an unused room, little attention needs to be paid to its appearance and an old refrigerator can be converted into a climate-controlled chamber. However, if it is to stand in the living room, you might wish to build or have it built to match with your furniture. Sometimes an old piece of furniture can be refurbished with a bit of skill and effort, or a new matching piece can be bought and adapted. It is also practical and inconspicuous to store dry breeding setups in a cabinet. Make sure the heating and lights do not get too hot and are attached at a safe distance from the panels. Daily opening guarantees adequate ventilation, but it is safer to add one or two mesh-covered ventilation holes, if sawing holes into the furniture is an option.
Breeding setups can be kept in basements; to save energy; this is suitable primarily for setups that do not require high temperatures. In a large apartment with a separate room for vivariums and food animals, a whole shelf can be reserved for breeding setups. Those who live in their own house have it easiest. A separate space for breeding food animals is likely to be available, be it a room, an annex, or a

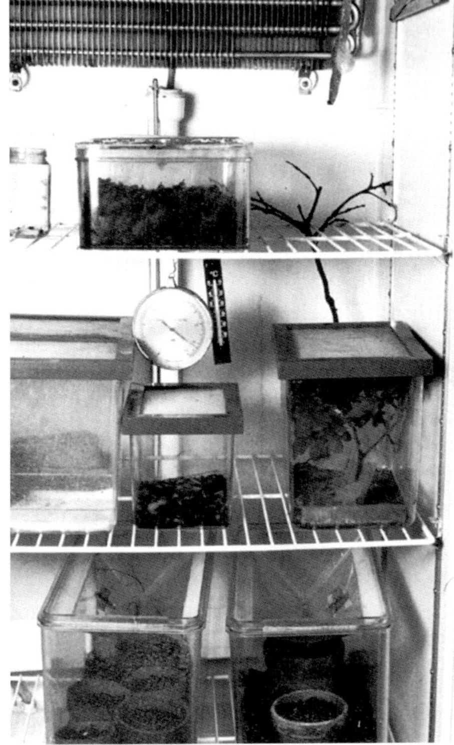

Fig. 4 View into a commercially available climate-controlled chamber.

greenhouse than can be heated to the required temperature. The warmth in the boiler room can also be exploited for breeding setups.

Breeding Food Animals

The food animals in this book—discussed in the order in which they appear systematically—have been selected according to the following criteria:

1. A setup must be viable for several generations. This is why mosquito larvae and black beetles (genus *Blaps*) are not included.
2. The breeding setup requires only a moderate amount of work, and the labor investment must be reasonable for the expected yield. This is why the *Helix pomatia* snail, night crawlers, and silkworms are missing.
3. The breeding process must be controllable and workable without damage to human food and furniture. This is why grain moths, rice flour beetles, some types of cockroaches, and mites are excluded.
4. The breeding of water snails, guppies, guinea pigs, rabbits, and other animals are not included because they are extensively described in other books and their use is limited to certain vivarium animals.
5. Some breeding instructions were kept in this edition of the book even though these animals have not been kept for a considerable time. This includes the Japanese water flea, and the two species of migratory locusts from South America and Morocco. This is to encourage interested parties to reestablish breeding colonies of these animals.

Plankton

What is plankton? The term "plankton" is a commonly used term that does not indicate a specific group of plants or animals. All aquatic organisms that have none or limited ability for independent movement are included. If they are plants they are called phytoplankton, if they are of animal origin they are called zooplankton. To add a certain amount of organization to all the included organisms, they are categorized by their size. Organisms smaller than 0.05 mm are called nanoplankton, those between 0.05 and 0.2 mm microplankton, and those larger macroplankton. It is easy to imagine that each group contains a large variety of shapes and forms of organisms. Primary plankton organisms are green algae, flagellates, ciliates, and bacteria. Sometimes the term infusoria (lat. infusum) is used (because of their occurrence in infusions; that is, organic substances that are covered with water and left to stand, as for example hay, straw, lettuce, or dirt). Of course, the species that are relevant in freshwater aquarium science are different from those in marine aquarium science. Plankton is essential for raising fish fry, because these small organisms can be eaten from the first day, before larger prey like brine shrimp can be offered. It is beyond this book to cover the extensive topic of keeping and breeding plankton with all its challenges and problems. It

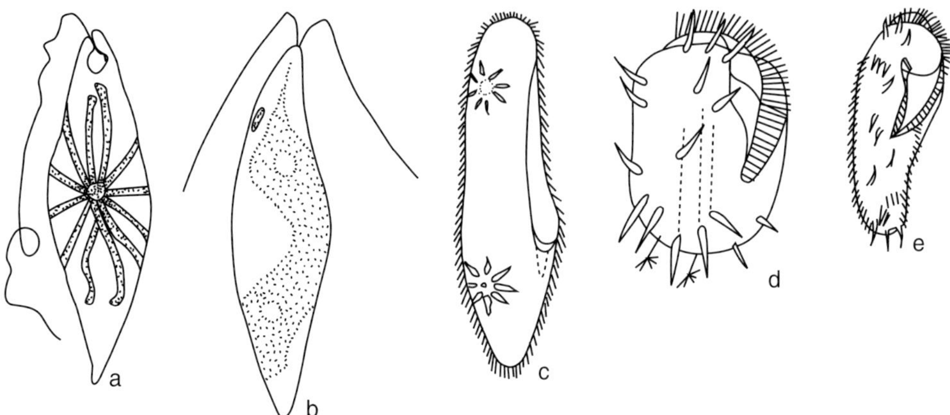

Fig. 5 Examples of single-cell organisms: a) *Euglena viridis*, b) *Chlorogonium*, c) the ciliate *Paramecium caudatum*, d) *Euplotes patella*, e) *Stylonychia mutilus*.

only provides some useful hints and tricks. If you wish to dig deeper and would like to delve into this material more intensely, refer to the list of references with books on the many methods for breeding and keeping food animals.

Containers and sterilization: The breeding containers and their sterilization deserve some attention so that the setups can be kept at least partially sterile. Unrefined cultures can be kept in ordinary glass and plastic containers like those found in any household. For pure cultures, it is preferable to use tools and containers made from Jena glass; this is a matter of course if you need to boil and sterilize them. To cultivate food algae, including single-celled ones like *Paramecium*, plastic petri dishes have proven suitable.

To breed larger quantities of saltwater plankton, Plexiglas or glass tanks from 20 l and up are suitable; they need not be sterilized.

None of the tools and containers should contain poisonous substances or come in contact with metal (copper, brass).

For simple sterilization, close the beaker or retort with aluminum foil and bake it in the oven at a temperature of about 100°C. Be careful with plastic bowls—they usually deform. All glass containers should be rinsed well with distilled, or if unavailable, demineralized, water.

Freshwater Plankton

Freshwater plankton (Fig. 5) is relatively easy to acquire, either with a small plankton net from any body of standing water, or by making an infusion. Sometimes an old aquarium filter will produce a good yield. To catch plankton you need a net and pint-size sealable plastic bottles, or even plastic bags. The net is made of very fine mesh. At the tapered end of the net is small removable cup. To fish for plankton, the net is slowly dragged through the water several times, then the contents of the cup are emptied into a container for transport; it is only filled halfway so that breathing air is available.

Only water from the same place where the plankton was caught may be used; tap water is deadly. Since some organisms are sensitive to heat, it is recommended to transport the bottles in a cooler.

Such acquired material is called an unrefined culture; it contains a variety of organisms. Take water from the same place where the plankton was collected and fill large bottling jars or small (10-20 l) glass aquariums (full glass) and add a small amount of the collected plankton. Pour everything over an artemia net to get rid of impurities and larger organisms.

If the mix contains many green algae, place the jars in a bright location. Avoid direct sunlight. Cover the jars with glass lids to keep out dust. With this setup, the plankton will stay alive for days or even weeks, and it may even reproduce. These unrefined cultures form the basis for pure cultures.

Infusions: This section discusses infusions and easy-to-keep pure cultures. Following these guidelines, many single-celled organisms can be bred with little effort. This is done using a medium that serves as food for bacteria that then serve as food for the infusoria. These infusions can be created using a variety of organic materials. The best known is an infusion made with hay, but infusoria can also be made by covering a leaf of lettuce or a piece of banana peel with water and letting it sit for a few days. These infusions and the ones described below use small amounts of materials that are removed completely after a few days.

To start a large culture of *Paramecium caudatum*, slices of rutabaga (not sugar beet!) are extremely good. A piece of rutabaga is cubed and dried in the sun or with a heater. Avoid high temperatures during drying. The dry pieces will keep in a sealed can for a long time. Fill a jar with 200-300 ml of water from a pond or fishtank and add 1-2 pieces of rutabaga. In sequence, a large number of bacteria will develop in this setup; first small ciliates, and after 8-14 days a large number of the ciliate *Paramecium caudatum*. Continue as follows: A wide-necked Erlenmeyer flask is loosely filled with straw and filled with tap water until the straw is covered. Then, to achieve partial sterilization, the whole assembly is brought to a boil. After cooling, it is inoculated with *Paramecium caudatum* from the rutabaga setup. If you succeed in transplanting only *Paramecium caudatum*, then you have already an almost pure culture. After only a few days so many *Paramecium caudatum* develop that the water appears cloudy. They can be harvested using a pipette, strained over nylon gauze (30 μm) and used as food. These kinds of cultures remain viable for months, and kept at a temperature of 15-18°C they produce a good number of animals continuously.

Occasionally the setup has to be topped off with boiled tap water. Feeding is not necessary. The top of the jar should be covered with glass or a cotton ball to prevent infection with other bacteria. Depending on need, a whole rack of jars can be kept.

This method can be used to cultivate other organisms as well that eat bacteria. Such cultures can also be kept in the dark, and if they cannot be attended to for an extended period, they can be stored in the refrigerator.

Milk culture: *Paramecium caudatum* and Stentoridae can be cultivated in milk. Add one drop of milk to 200-500 ml of boiled water. Add another drop of milk after a few days. Once the solution is completely clear, inoculate it with *Paramecium caudatum*. This causes a population explosion after which the culture has to be moved into a fresh cultivation medium; that is, new milk/water solution.

Dirt-Cheese Culture: Ongoing cultures of *Euglena gracilis* can be created by using dirt and hard cheese. Cover the bottom of an Erlenmeyer flask (100-250 ml) with dirt, add a lentil-size piece of hard-cheese, and cover with sand (dirt and sand must not contain fertilizers). Fill the flask to ¾ with tap water. Use cotton wool or cellulose to close the top. Put the flask into a pot of water and boil for about one hour. After cooling, inoculate with a few milliliters from an existing *Euglena* culture. Place the culture in a bright location (Euglenas contain chlorophyll!). After a while, about a week, the water starts to turn light green, then dark green and opaque. This continues for a while until the number of cells decreases noticeably. Start a new culture before this stage is reached. Euglenas are tough: Should the culture ever dry out, it can be restarted simply by adding water. These cultures can also be grown using a dirt solution only, and it is recommended to keep a small amount of dirt solution handy in the refrigerator. Proceed similarly as with the dirt-cheese method: Boil equal parts of dirt and water for one hour. After cooling off, run through a filter and sterilize for about an hour. Since an autoclave (a high-pressure apparatus where heating beyond the boiling point is possible) is not usually available, a pressure cooker can be employed to boil the water at high pressure. If an autoclave

is available, sterilize at 120°C for about 20 minutes. This concentrated solution keeps for months in the refrigerator. To use it, dilute it with tap water that has been standing for a while (to evaporate the chlorine); use 2-5 ml of the dirt solution for each 100 ml of water.

Cultures Using Inorganic Nutrient Solution: Trading more effort for better results the cultivation media can be created directly from stock solutions. These stock solutions can be used for ciliates like *Euplotes*, *Stylonychia*, and many more. The Pringsheim method has proven its value.

Do the following: Fill four clean glass or plastic bottles with 1 liter of boiled and if possible demineralized water; then add:

Bottle I   4 g Dinatrium hydrogen phosphate
             $Na_2HPO_4 \cdot 2\ H_2O$
Bottle II   4 g Magnesium sulfate
             $Mg\ SO_4 \cdot 7H_2O$
Bottle III 40 g Calcium nitrate – 4-hydrate
             $Ca\ (NO)_2 \cdot 4\ H_2O$
Bottle IV 5.2 g Potassium chloride KCl
             + 10 ml salicid acid 1 n HCl

(The amounts indicated must be followed precisely.)

For use as a medium, 15 ml from each of these solutions must be added to 3 liters of boiled and demineralized water. The algae needed as food for many cultures (similar to *Euglena*) as for example *Chlorogonium*, can be cultured in Pringsheim or dirt solutions. It must be emphasized again that regardless of the cultivation medium the cultures must be transferred into a fresh medium regularly.

Creating Pure Cultures: Up until now, the discussion has focused on unrefined and simple permanent cultures. We did mention more or less pure cultures that contain exclusively or almost exclusively one type of organism. They can be produced; however, this requires some skill and experience, and a few additional tools. Indispensable are binoculars or a simple microscope, several glass dishes of various sizes, some glass piping, pipettes, and a small petroleum burner.

The easiest purification method is the dilution method. A few drops are taken from the unrefined culture, placed on a slide, and examined under the binoculars. If the desired type of organism shows up in large numbers, one drop is moved from the slide to a small dish or to another slide and diluted again with a small amount of culture medium. This is repeated until only one type of organism can be found.

Then the animals are moved to a prepared, relatively small culture container. At first, they must be fed carefully; just a few drops are sufficient. Soon the single-celled organisms will have reproduced enough that more food can be offered. Foods are milk or food algae. After a few days, the culture must be transferred and it is possible to work with larger containers now.

With the next method, the desired single-celled organism is transferred from the unrefined culture into the culture medium by means of a capillary pipette. This requires some practice and will not work the first time. Observe a sample under the binoculars, guide the pipette over the animal to catch, and dip the pipette into the drop. The capillary force will suction up water and the animal. The same can also be accomplished by connecting the end of the pipette to a hose. Put the hose in your mouth and by sucking at the appropriate moment the desired single-celled organism can be caught.

Such extremely thin capillary pipettes (external diameter 0.5-1 mm) can be purchased from laboratory supply stores. The captured organisms are examined again in a small amount of medium to make sure no undesirable animals are part of the mix. Finally, they are transferred to the cultivation medium to start a pure culture.

Ocean Plankton

Compared to freshwater aquarium science, plankton plays an even larger role in saltwater aquarium science. In the former, only fish fry feed on plankton, while the most interesting saltwater organisms are those that feed on plankton. Most of these can only be fed, and under ideal conditions bred, on living plankton.

The methods used for working with freshwater plankton can largely be adopted, with the difference that exclusively ocean water is used. Ocean plankton is much more sensitive, especially to increases in temperature, and they require more oxygen. Only a few forms out of a large variety can be cultivated.

This includes the saltwater form of *Euplotes* and the rotifer *Brachionus*. Sized at 5-10 µm (*Euplotes*) and 30-60 µm (*Brachionus*) they offer a suitable sequence of food for raising marine fish, which can be followed by nauplius larvae and brine shrimp.

Food algae, like *Dunaliella salina* and the *Chlorella* species can be bred easily. Breeding stock can be acquired from saltwater tanks that are overgrown with algae. The algae can be scraped from the glass, or water can be drawn from near the glass. Since ocean salt is rather expensive, being frugal with it is usually desirable. For breeding plankton, water that is siphoned from a saltwater tank during a routine water change is perfectly suitable. However, if medication has been added to the water recently, it is unusable for breeding plankton. Before using the water, filter over Perlon filter wool to remove mud and dirt particles.

Breeding algae requires a seawater-dirt solution. It is prepared in the same way as described for freshwater plankton; of course, saltwater is used instead of freshwater. The finished concentrate is diluted (about 2-5 ml of dirt solution for each 100 ml of saltwater) to produce a medium for *Dunaliella* and *Chlorella* (further instructions see *Euglena gracilis*).

Euplotes and *Brachionus* are fed with algae, baking yeast solution, a trace of squashed *Tubifex* worms or ground meat. The bacteria that grow from this will serve as food. Ideal, because it is clean, Preis-Microplan, a commercially available invertebrate food, is one without problems. If it is used according to the manufacturer's instructions, breeding the plankton is possible without difficulty. The best results with *Euplotes* and *Brachionus* are achieved by growing them in pure or mixed cultures. Pure cultures are preferred since otherwise the *Euplotes* get the upper hand and the *Brachionus* disappear. Both of these planktons tolerate variations in the salt concentration. Only the water temperature must be adjusted during transfer. The ideal breeding temperature is 22-24°C. Containers with *Euplotes* and *Crachionus* should not be exposed to direct sunlight; a small amount of brightness suffices. In a room that receives natural daylight, the breeding setups do not require artificial light.

Large-scale Breeding of *Euplotes* and *Brachionus*: These two types of plankton can easily be raised in large quantities. It is convenient to set up three 20 l breeding tanks that are filled once a week with saltwater from the aquarium and injected with algae from the container that was set up last. Each tank must be aerated with a kieselguhr (porous diatomite) aerator. The amount of air is calibrated so that no foam forms at the surface. For better air exchange, the tanks are not covered. The preferred food is Preis-Microplan because the water remains clear. To harvest plankton it can simply be skimmed off; it is always taken from the longest-running tank. After 3 weeks the remaining culture from the first tank is poured into a jar and the breeding tank is cleaned carefully with clear water and a sponge. It is refilled with saltwater and the saved "solution" which now serves as seed water is added. A week later, the second tank is cleaned, and so forth.

Lange and Kaiser (1989) describe their process for a continuing breeding setup that they developed at the Berlin zoo-aquarium: "The complete plankton cultivation takes place in 28 full glass tanks of 300 liters. The tanks have valves at the bottom for emptying them during cleaning. To start a culture, the thoroughly cleaned tanks are filled with 30 cm of saltwater that has twice as much salt as ocean water, inoculated with 10 liters of algae culture and illuminated with an 80-watt HQL lamp (high intensity pressurized mercury) lamp for 24 hours. Because of the high salt concentration, all the zooplankton dies off while the phytoplankton develops. When the phytoplankton culture, stored at 26-30°C, shows a light green color after 4-7 days, the tank is filled up to 60 cm with warmed up tap water to reach the normal salt concentration. At the same time, the tank is aerated and inoculated with zooplankton. The zooplankton reproduces fast and can soon be harvested with a plankton net for use as food.

Accessories and Breeding Stock: Much of what is required to breed plankton is commercially available and should be quite useful as a starting point. There is "plankton substitute," a liquid algae suspension that also contains rotifers, ciliates and many other types of plankton. In addition, natural, frozen, and even living ocean plankton is available.

For the completely inexperienced, infusoria granules (Protogen-Granulat) can be useful. These are concentrates of dried infusoria that only need to be sprinkled into the aquarium to grow live plankton. From these, cultures can be established and pure cultures can be isolated.

Breeding stock for single-celled organisms like *Euplotes, Stylonychia, Paramecium,* and others can usually be acquired from microbiological and zoological institutes. They might also be available from experienced aquarium enthusiasts who have their own setups; this is where local clubs can be useful. The required glass containers and filters can be bought at any laboratory supply store.

Feeding: When feeding plankton to vivarium animals consider that most of these cultures contain some decayed materials; accumulating too much of these substances in the aquarium water should be avoided. It helps to filter the food over nylon gauze first. Use a fine fabric with a mesh size of about 30 µm, which will retain most single-celled organisms. The gauze with the attached organisms is rinsed in the tank. If the sample only needs to be separated from larger particles or animals, gauze with a mesh size of 90-118 µm can be used. Single-celled organisms easily pass through this mesh. Only pure cultures of ocean plankton can be used directly without any precautions. Freshwater tank enthusiasts consider plankton the best first food for baby fish. It is also useful for breeding water fleas and brine shrimp.

For saltwater tanks, the use of plankton extends to all plankton-eating organisms, including coral, tube worms, young sea needles and sea horses, clams, sponges, prawns, and others.

Advantages and Disadvantages:

Advantages:

- Unproblematic first food for all young fish
- Seasonally independent if kept in a place where no freezing occurs
- Most natural food for breeding *Artemia (Dunaliella)*

Disadvantages:

- Beginners must gain some experience
- Pretty large investment in time and equipment
- Requires extremely clean work habits
- Neglected cultures smell bad

Nematodes (Round Worms)

Among Nemathelminthes, the nematodes are by far the largest class with more than

10,000 species. They are round, string-shaped, usually long worms that live either independently (in the ground) or as parasites. Free-living nematodes are usually rather small, and so are the kinds that are known as food animals. They belong to the genus *Turbatrix* (=*Anguillula*) within the family of the Cephalobidae, order Rhabditoidea (= Anguilluloidea).

Vinegar Eels
(*Turbatrix silusiae* and *Turbatrix aceti*)

Distinguishing between the various species is difficult and not important for the vivarium enthusiast. The male eels reach about 1 mm, the females 2-2.5 mm, and rarely, under optimal conditions, 4 mm. The gender ratio is 1:2, and the babies are 0.2 mm long when they are born. These worms live in fermenting bacterial substances. The transparent animals can barely be seen with the naked eye. The body is long and stretched out, round, and covered with a rough skin. Their common name derives from their looks and from the way they move like eels. They lack eyes; food is sucked in.

Development times: The female worms are ovoviviparous (that is, the egg contains a fully developed young animal) and give birth to up to 45 young 5 days after fertilization. In 10 days, the young females become sexually mature, the males about a day later. The animals live for about 45 days, but it is said they can survive for up to 10 months. The little eels multiply extremely fast. At a temperature of 18-20°C Knaack counted 25,000 animals in 1 ml of nutrient solution. After 10 days, there were 130,000!

Containers, Cultivation Medium, and Setup: Shallow pickling jars, petri dishes, shallow plastic containers or similar containers with a footprint of 50-100 cm^2 are suitable. Depending on the breeding method, these cultures will develop a more or less strong odor, depending on whether they can be kept open or covered. A cover is recommended to avoid infestation with fruit flies.

Two breeding methods have been used successfully. For the first, leached out coffee grounds are poured into a container to a level of about 2 cm and enough beer is added to barely cover the coffee grounds. For the second method the eels live in mush that is filled in to a height of 1-2 cm.

Food: When using the coffee grounds method, the sole food for the worms is the beer or brewer's yeast paste. When the culture dries out, a little bit of water is added. The paste for the second method is prepared from oats or gruel mixed up cold with milk or water to a thick consistency. According to Essmann (1986), "Alete-6-Korn" or "Milupa-7-Korn" porridge is mixed with a little baking yeast until it forms a big lump. Adding the yeast reduces the strong to nauseating smell considerably that the breeding container emits after a while, an experience that Sterzel (1989) also reports. Another recipe (Knaack, 1958) requires mixing enough hot water with wheat flour until it turns to a thick paste. After it cools, it is inoculated with worms. However, in this last food the worms will not crawl up the walls of the container so that separating them from their cultivation medium is rather involved. If gruel is used as the medium, it is not necessary to provide additional foods; however, after a while, baking yeast, oatmeal, or wheat cereal can be added.

Notes: Breeding these nematodes is simple and cannot go wrong. A teaspoon of breeding stock is dropped into the prepared jar. The eels multiply in a very short time and can be harvested after a few days. A setup remains viable for about a month. Even if the worms are not being harvested, the setups must be checked every couple of weeks as it is possible for them to spoil or be infested by fungi of mites. Depending on the required amounts, it is enough to start a new setup every month, or they can be started at regular intervals, for example weekly, so that there are always worms available.

Feeding: The adult worms crawl up the sides of their container and sit above the cultivation medium in a thick layer. From there they can be harvested using a small piece of wood, a shaving blade, or a soft brush.

Once dropped into the aquarium, they sink slowly to the bottom and remain alive for up to 48 hours (Rössel, 1988) in freshwater. For surface-feeding fish, a feeding ring can be lined with the finest nylon gauze and the worms placed on top. They will slowly escape toward the bottom where they can be caught by the fish. They also wiggle around at the bottom of the tank for a while where they are available to catfish, cichlids, and barbs. To avoid an undesired buildup of bacteria in the aquarium, make sure that no large amounts of dead worms remain in the tank.

Microworms are a good fish food, especially for raising babies. They are not just used for freshwater aquariums but more and more often for saltwater tanks, too.

Pests and Diseases: Do not allow mold to develop; if necessary, start a new setup.

Advantages and Disadvantages:

Advantage:
- Requires little space and upkeep

Disadvantages:
- May smell after a time
- Fat content too high to use as sole food for raising fish

Segmented Worms (Annelids)

As the name "segmented worms" suggests, the long-stretched, usually completely round body of the Annelids is made up of many segments. These do not just appear as ridges on the outside, but are also reflected in the inner structuring of the organs. They are thus easily distinguished from the nematodes. The segments are arranged almost uniformly between the prostomium with the mouth opening and the posterior tip with the anus. Each segment has bundles of bristles (setae), and the polychete worms that live in the ocean have fleshy, lateral outgrowths (parapodia) that represent a first indication of extremities. Annelids can be found in the oceans, freshwater, and the ground; some live as parasites. The terrestrial annelids are easiest to breed, in particular the representatives of two families, the Enchytraeidae and the Lumbriculidae (includes earthworms). Both families belong to the order of the Oligochaeta, which has about 2400 species. Together with the leeches, they belong to the class Clitellata that also includes earthworms. The clitellum, which gives this group its name, forms a ring-shaped tube covering several segments in the first third of the body. The secretions that its glands produce play a role in worm mating and forming the cocoon for the eggs.

Clitellata are hermaphrodites, which means they produce both eggs as well as sperm. Like snails, during mating sperm is exchanged and both animals lay fertile eggs. The eggs hatch either into larvae or—for Clitellata—small worms. They have only a few segments. They have a growth zone near the tail, where more segments form later.

White Worms
(*Enchytraeus albidus*)
Grindal Worms
(*Enchytraeus buchholzi*)

Description: The Enchytraeus family includes about 20 different species some-times with different requirements. They live in moist, loose dirt, compost heaps, and even flower pots, where they feed in the same way as earthworms and thus change the composition of the dirt simi-larly. Interesting for the vivarium enthusi-ast are two species in particular, because they are easy to breed.

Enchytraeus albidus is a 20-36 mm long small, whitish worm with a diameter of about 0.5–0.75 mm.

Enchytraeus buchholzi is closely related to the former but smaller, about 5-10 mm long, and prefers higher temperatures. It is very possible that common cultures also contain other species, but this is not relevant for breeding purposes.

Development Times: Precise data on development and reproduction times for the two *Enchytraeus* species are not known to the authors.

Containers, Substrate, and Setups:
Enchytraeus albidus: The best breeding container is a shallow wooden box with a rim about 15 cm high. For a cover, use fine gauze or a similarly meshed fabric nailed to a frame that is slightly larger than the box's circumference. In this way, pests can pretty much be kept out. There is no need to be picky about breeding containers; flower pots or shallow clay trays are also suitable. Metal cans are not recommended because they rust and the dirt easily gets too wet and lumpy, especially since cans have a small surface area. All containers are set up on small blocks or pieces of wood so that the air can circulate underneath. Those who require large amounts of worms should set up multiple cultures, so that a single culture is not weakened by overharvesting. By alternating from which culture worms are harvested, there should always be plenty available.

Any loose, unfertilized dirt makes a suitable substrate. Potting soil, improved with forest soil and sifted sand for aeration should be ideal. Mixing in some peat moss (unfertilized!) can only be advantageous, because it keeps the dirt lose and at the same time regulates the humidity. Soils that contain clay are not suitable; they get easily lumpy and the surface forms a crust when it dries out, which causes the worms to die from lack of air. The substrate is kept moist but not wet throughout the lifetime of the setup, and it must remain loose and porous. Should the dirt get too wet by accident, this can be remedied by adding some sawdust.

Fill the dirt mixture loosely into the prepared container. Make an indentation in the middle for placing the food. Add the seed worms on top and lightly cover them with 1-2 cm of dirt. Cover the container with a piece of large-meshed fabric, for example sackcloth, and wet it all with a gentle moistening from a watering can. It is often recommended to cover the indentation for the food with a glass pane. However, this limits airflow and can be a disadvantage. If in doubt, try both methods and use the one that works better.

After running the setup for a longer period of time, the substrate must be renewed. To this end, the dirt is allowed to dry out slowly. The worms will stay in the humid areas, abandon the walls of the container, and clump up in the middle. The ball of worms can be removed and transferred to a new container.

Enchytraeus buchholzi: Breeding grindal worms follows more or less the same procedure as breeding the ordinary *Enchytraeus*. Large flower pots or bowls have proven to be good breeding containers. A volume of 2 l suffices. Grindal worms prefer almost pure peat moss (unfertilized) that is mixed with a small amount of fine sand. This substrate is arranged loosely in the intended breeding container. Of course, a lid must be used to close it off. The pot is moistened thoroughly and the worms are added.

Food: *Enchytraeus albidus*: There are numerous recipes and options and there are no limits to the joys of experimentation in this area. The worms will often refuse to eat what is offered and one is forced to try out other foods. One of the most proven recipes is to moisten oats with a little water or milk and add maybe a trace of sugar and a little bit of margarine. This paste, which must not be liquid, is spooned into the prepared indentation in the dirt of the breeding container. If the feeding paste is too watery, it will leech into the dirt, go sour, and spoil, which is harmful. Cooked oats, mash for laying hens softened with boiling water, or soft, unsalted, even raw vegetable garbage (fruit pies, spinach, lettuce) can be fed. Densely populated setups can also be fed a small amount of raw egg; however, care must be taken that it is consumed within two days. In all cases food should be portioned in such a way that all of it is consumed within a few days. Any spoiled food must be removed completely and immediately.

Enchytraeus buchholzi: To feed this worm, dry oats are simply sprinkled onto the surface of the substrate. Do not overfeed! The oats must not be allowed to develop mold. The available food should be eaten within a day.

If there are too many worms in the setup, the substrate will usually start to smell. At this time it is best to start up a new breeding container.

Breeding Conditions: Once the breeding container is prepared and seeded with worms in the described fashion, it is placed in a dark location where the white worms grow best at a temperature of almost 18°C. Grindal worms need higher temperatures for fast reproduction, around 18-24°C. If the temperature drops to 13°C, the reproduction ceases. It is therefore necessary to check regularly on the temperature. If they are kept at their preferred temperature, grindal worms breed faster than white worms.

Both species can be exposed to temperatures as low as 4°C without being damaged, however, reproduction ceases.

About 3 weeks after starting the breeding

setups, the worms can be harvested and fed to vivarium animals; by then the breeding container should be full of worms. The dirt must stay moist and crumbly; wet and lumpy dirt inhibits reproduction.

Pests: To prevent infestation with pests, a few simple rules must be followed when cultivating *Enchytraeus* worms. If too much food is offered, or food remains in the container for too long, mites will appear quickly.

Sometimes, however, they are introduced with the first inoculation. When the surface of the substrate is inspected with a magnifying glass, many brownish or whitish small balls can be seen. These are definitely not worm eggs but mites. To fight the mites naturally, a few woodlice can be introduced (they can be found in any basement or in the yard under rocks and flower pots). They do not harm the worms but will busily devour the mites. However, if mites appear in masses, stronger remedies are required. Cover a glass pane with grease or another sticky substance and place it inside the breeding container. After a relatively short time, about 1-2 days, mites will stick to it. They can then be removed. After doing this repeatedly, the setup will be free of mites.

Much more dangerous, because they can destroy whole breeding setups, are small, 2 mm long, black *ichneumon* wasps. At first glance, they look like small flies. In their customary ways, they pierce the worms' skin and lay their eggs inside their bodies. The hatching wasp larvae eat the *Enchytraeus* worms. Here, too, a sticky, nonpoisonous substance comes handy. Attach a piece of cardboard or a sheet of paper under the lid and cover it with the sticky paste. The *ichneumon* wasps get stuck and can be removed. This method requires a tightly closing lid, which also prevents renewed infestation. Continue this procedure until the last wasp remaining in the substrate has hatched.

When too much food is present, it will attract bluebottle flies, whose larvae can decimate the worms. They are especially attracted to raw egg leftovers. Once a breeding setup is infested, the top layer of the substrate must be replaced with every feeding. In general, it is good advice to destroy a setup after it has been infested and start from scratch.

Feeding: The worms often congregate around the feeding area so densely, that they can be removed in almost pure form. If this is not the case, and food or dirt sticks to them, they can be dropped into a small bowl of water. After a short time, the worms will form a tight ball, become clean, and are usable as food. To feed fish, the worms are placed in a feeding sieve from which they are pulled by the fish. For fish that preferably or exclusively feed at the bottom, a ball of worms is dropped into a small glass bowl, which is placed on the bottom of the aquarium. In this way, the worms cannot escape into the substrate and remain available to the fish. If the worms are too large for the baby fish, they could conceivably be chopped finely with a razor or squashed. In general, it is not recommended to feed fish exclusively on *Enchytraeus* worms. The fish can easily get too fat, their colors will fade, and they will breed less readily; even infertility is possible. The worms are recommended as a supplemental food, however.

Land-dwelling amphibians receive the worms in small bowls, slightly moistened, so that they do not dry out.

In addition to all freshwater fish, lizards, frogs, toads and salamanders also like *Enchytraeus* worms. They are also useful for raising water turtles. Furthermore, they can be offered to all tadpoles of frogs as well as crayfish, anemones, and starfish. As a supplemental food, they are also suitable for water shrews and spiny anteaters. Care must be taken when feeding the worms to tropical saltwater fish, as they are not suitable for all species.

Delicate insect-eating song birds, for example, the Chiffchaff and other warblers, Old World warblers, robins, but also tropical species, like *Enchytraeus* worms. They are offered in bowls mixed with a small amount of clean dirt. This has the advantage that the birds will eat dirt, which is rich in minerals and trace elements, together with the worms.

Advantages and Disadvantages:

Advantages:
- Needs little room and small amount of upkeep
- If done right, the setups are odor free

Disadvantages:
- Often infested with mites
- Because of the high fat content, only suitable as supplemental food

Red Marsh Worms or Red Wrigglers (*Lumbricus rubellus*) Redworms or Compost Worms (*Eisenia foetida*) *Dendrobaena* Earthworms (*Dendrobaena* spec.)

Description: To look at earthworms as food for vivarium animals covers a small excerpt from a large chapter. Not only are

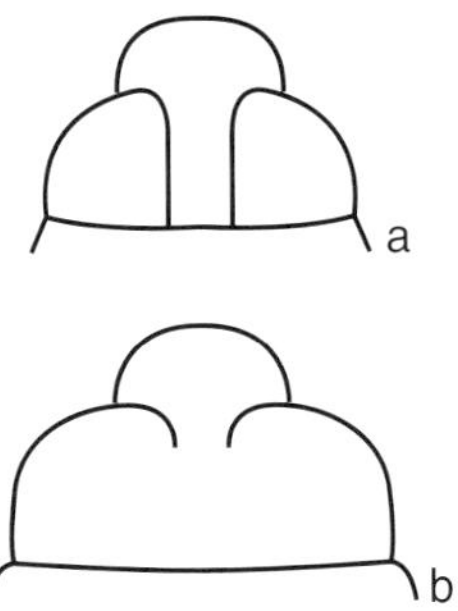

Fig. 6 Prostomium of earthworms. a) Red wriggler (*Lumbricus rubellus*), b) redworm (*Eisenia foetida*).

the number of earthworms that are used as fishing bait significant, but their metabolic by-products are even more important than they themselves are: Worm casts are the foundation for the fertility of soils almost worldwide. Those who are interested in worm composting can refer to a small but excellent book by Walter Buch (1986).

Lumbricus rubellus: (Fig. 8) Red marsh worms or red wrigglers reach a stretched out length of 12-15 cm and are about 5 mm in diameter. Their body is round with a flattened tail. The back is brown red, the skin shimmers purple-iridescent, and the underside shows a light grey-brown coloration. The clitellum lies over the 26th 32nd segments. If looked at from above with a strong magnifying glass, the prostomium divides the following segment completely (see Fig. 6a) in all *Lumbricus* species.

The yellow-green cocoon is egg-shaped, 3-4 mm long and 2-2.5 mm in diameter. The whitish, thread-thin young worms measure 8-10 mm at when they hatch.

Eisenia foetida: (Fig. 7) The redworm remains at 10-13 cm length and 3-4 mm

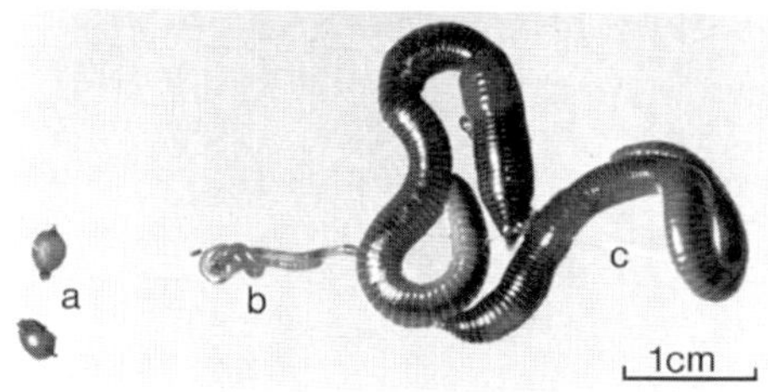

Fig. 7 Redworm (*Eisenia foetida*). a) Egg cocoon, b) young worms, c) sexually mature adults.

diameter a little smaller. It is colored wine or brown-red all around with yellow segmental lines. The prostomium does not completely divide the following segment (Fig. 6b).
After hatching from a lemon-shaped cocoon the young are 5-8 mm long and whitish transparent.
Dendrobaena sp.: This muscular type of worm reaches a size of 13-16 cm and has a 6-7 mm diameter. On top it is brown red; at the head, near the clitellum pretty dark, then lighter with a darker stripe along the center; segmental lines are lighter. The underside is paler and yellowish toward the tail. The body is flattened in shape. Cocoon and hatchlings are the same as *Lumbricus rubellus*. This worm supposedly originates in the United States, but the species has not been determined exactly.
The ordinary garden earthworm (*Lumbricus terrestris*) is less suitable for breeding. It requires a container that is at least 25 cm deep, flees at the slightest disturbance, and produces only about 50 offspring per year; breeding this worm is therefore not discussed here.
Development Cycle: When fed well, all three kinds of worms reproduce easily.

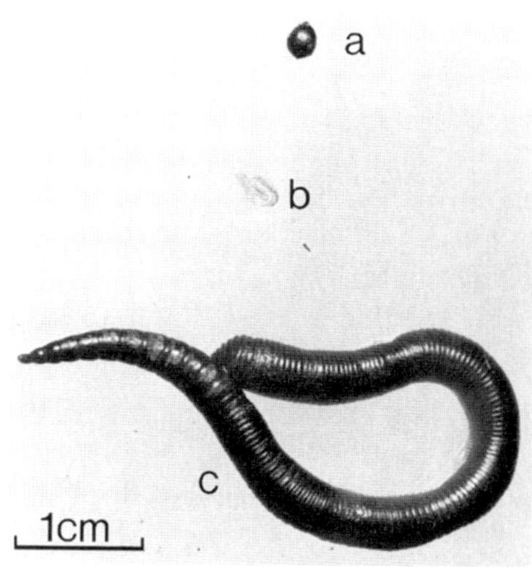

Fig. 8 Red wriggler (*Lumbricus rubellus*). a) Egg cocoon, b) young worms, c) sexually mature adult.

Each animal lays about 2 cocoons per week. Each cocoon contains 2-4, sometimes up to 8 eggs that hatch after about 10 days. This makes for about 350-450 expected offspring per worm per year. Worms start to reproduce at about 3 months of age.
Containers, Substrate, and Equipment: Any container that has a tight-fitting lid, is at least 25 cm high, and tolerates humidity, is suitable, including buckets, storage boxes, Styrofoam chests, wooden boxes, etc. It is advantageous to have small holes at the bottom to drain excess water (if one is careful to prevent accumulation of standing water at the bottom, the holes are not necessary). A container that measures 40 x 30 x 25 cm can house, depending on the species, 100-2000 worms.
If a yard is available, a wooden pen can be prepared, measuring about 150 x 80 cm

and 60 cm tall. To prevent the worms from escaping, the boards are dug 20 cm into the ground. Up to 20,000 worms can live in such an enclosure, provided the substrate is kept moist and plenty of food is provided.

The substrate is made up of equal parts of garden dirt (not potting soil!), and peat moss. To loosen it up, some coarse sand and leaf litter are mixed in. The latter is especially important for *Lumbricus rubellus*. The dirt mixture is moistened thoroughly and filled into the breeding container. To retain moisture, the dirt can be covered with foil in such a way that air can still enter into the substrate. Underneath the foil, a piece of sackcloth can be arranged in several layers as the worms like to crawl through it.

To keep the worms healthy, the substrate requires a pH of 5.5-6.5; that is, mildly acidic. If the dirt is too acidic (pH value below 5.5), it can be mixed with limestone or chalk powder. If the ph is above 7, that is, alkaline, the substrate can be moistened with a weak solution of vinegar and water.

Food: The earthworms are fed a diet of oats, coarsely ground corn, and other ground up grains that can be mixed with honey. In addition, greens like lettuce, carrot greens (Möller, 1954), cultivated and wild herbs, chopped up kitchen scraps, thin layers of lawn clippings, as well as finely grated vegetables and fruit: potatoes, carrots, apples. A small amount of food is placed in an indentation in the dirt, moistened, and covered again. Every 4-6 days the container should be inspected to see whether the food has been consumed, and new food should only be offered if all the old food has been consumed. Moldy food must be removed immediately. *Eisenia* and *Dendrobaena* will also eat table scraps.

Breeding Conditions:

Light: These light-sensitive worms remain in the dirt. Therefore, it does not matter whether the container is placed in a dark or light spot.

Heat: The worms start to breed at about 12°C. The temperature can rise to about 20°C. Higher temperatures are tolerated for short periods; *Dendrobaena* tolerates up to 30°C.

Humidity: Earthworms do not like standing water or dryness, therefore the substrate should be kept evenly moist.

Notes: After obtaining worms to stock your setup, simply place them on top of the dirt in the breeding container. Healthy animals will dig immediately into the substrate, while weak or dead animals remain on the top from where they can be collected after a while. Dead worms do not just smell bad, they also spoil the substrate.

To raise the worms sorted by size, several containers are required. To move the adults into a new container every 2 weeks, 7 containers are needed, for a 3-week cycle, 5 containers. When the dirt dries out, the worms clump up in balls. Since it is unwise to harm the cocoons and young worms by drying out the substrate, the adults must be sorted out by hand. In a large-scale breeding setup, the worms should always be sorted by size. If it is not important that worms of different sizes live side by side, and for limited requirements, one container suffices. However, then the container should not be stocked with too many worms such that there is plenty of room for the young worms, or adults should be harvested regularly to make room for offspring.

The *Eisenia foetida* worms that are harvested from compost heaps are known to smell bad and are only eaten after they have been washed. However, if they have been raised on grain and greens they can be fed directly out of their container. To remove worms from their container, only disturb the dirt in one place. Smaller worms can be found closer to the surface, often between leaves, large ones further down. If sackcloth is used to cover the dirt, worms can usually be found between the layers and harvested easily.

Storage: All worms can be stored for up to 4 weeks at 8°C, and up to 3 months at 2°C. For this purpose they are loosely packed into a breathable container like wood or Styrofoam in slightly moist dirt. Instead of dirt, soaked and stacked egg cartons can be used. Control humidity!

Pests and Diseases: Earthworms harbor parasites; however, they are usually no problem for the earthworms and never for the vivarium animals. However, the larvae of the flesh fly (*Sarcophaga carnaria*), which grow as parasites inside the earthworms, damage their hosts so much, that they do not survive.

Feeding: Fish, water turtles, and amphibians that live in the water can be fed directly with worms of the appropriate size. Take care that the worms are eaten before they can hide in the substrate. If only large worms are available, they can be cut up with a sharp knife or a razor blade. For land animals, the worms are offered in a bowl with a small amount of water.

Many animals love earthworms: fish, especially the larger species, frogs, toads, salamanders, and water turtles, many terrestrial lizards and many birds. Because of their calcium content, earthworms are a valuable source of food; they also trigger the hunting instinct, because they resist capture by wiggling.

Advantages and Disadvantages:
Advantages:
- Easy care
- Escaped animals do not cause damage
- Valuable, long-lived food animal

Disadvantages:
- Require relatively large amount space
- Dead animals stink terribly

Mollusks

The mollusks include such diverse animals as chitons, snails, squid, and shellfish. In the Gastropoda class (snails), the subclass pulmonate snails (Pulmonata) alone comprises over 20,000 known species. Thus it comes as no surprise that in the order Stylommatophora there are at least 3 terrestrial pulmonate snails with shells that are suitable for breeding. Representatives of the genus *Cepaea* belong to the family Helicidae, of the genus *Achatina* to the family Achatinidae.

Children are quite familiar with their shape. The snail crawls on its muscular foot over all obstacles. The head shows two pairs of stalks, the longer pair carries eyes on each tip, and they can be retracted like the fingers of a glove. The usually right-handed spiral shell consists of hardened calcium, which the snail enlarges in the course of its growth through secretions from its skin.

The snails discussed here are hermaphrodites. After mutual fertilization, they lay rather large eggs from which baby snails hatch complete with tiny shells.

Grove Snail
(*Cepaea nemoralis*)
Garden Snail
(*Cepaea hortensis*)

Description: *Cepaea nemoralis* (Fig. 9): The shell of the grove snail is spherical, somewhat wider than tall, and of a whitish to yellowish base color. Its height is 16-19 mm, its width 21-25 mm. Most specimens show 1-5 brown or black bands, occasionally animals without stripes are found. The umbilical area and labial palps are brown, the lips reddish brown or black. The dark gray body measures 3.5-4.5 cm when stretched out and is about 8 mm wide.

The white eggs, which are about 2.8-3.1 mm long and 2.3-2.6 mm thick have a calcified shell. The shell of the newborn snails is 2.7-2.9 mm wide. The grove snail can often be found in gardens, parks, and along train tracks, in shrubs, light woods, hills, and on walls. In the Alps it can be found to an altitude of 1300 m, in the Mittelgebirge until 600 m.

Cepaea hortensis (Fig. 10): The garden snail resembles the grove snail much. The shell is somewhat sturdier and smaller,

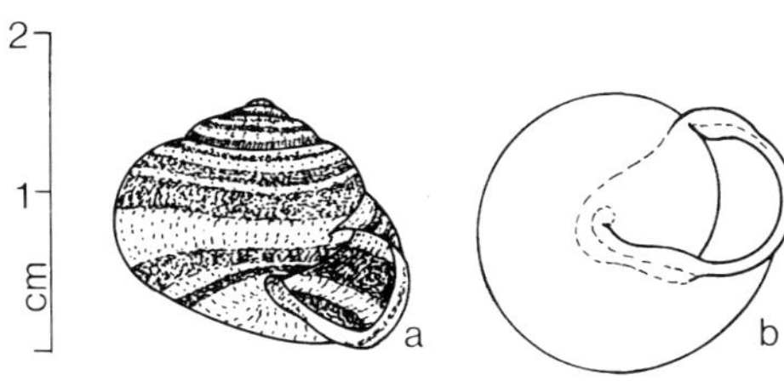
Fig. 10 Garden snail (*Cepaea hortensis*). a) Lateral view, b) ventral view.

14-16 mm tall and 19-21 mm wide. The quickest way to distinguish it from the grove snail is by the color of the lip of the aperture of the shell, the lip, and the umbilical area. These areas are white in the garden snail, sometimes pink. The color and size of the body are the same as for the grove snail.

The eggs and the young snails also resemble those of the grove snail. The garden snail inhabits bushes, light forests and hedges, rocks and walls; it is less often found in cultivated areas and can be found to higher altitudes than the grove snail, until 2000 m in the Alps and 750 m in the Mittelgebirge.

Development Cycles: The development of these snails occurs at a proverbial snail's pace: It takes them 12-18 months to complete their shell, and only then do they become sexually mature. The primary mating time starts after hibernation from about March to May. Each grove snail deposits 30-50 eggs three times between June and August. The snails hatch after 3-4 weeks. The garden snails usually produce 2 clutches of 30-60 eggs each that hatch after 2-2½ weeks. The hatchling snails weigh about 0.1 mg, about 3.4-4.5 g when grown. These numbers are for free-living snails according to Frömming (1954).

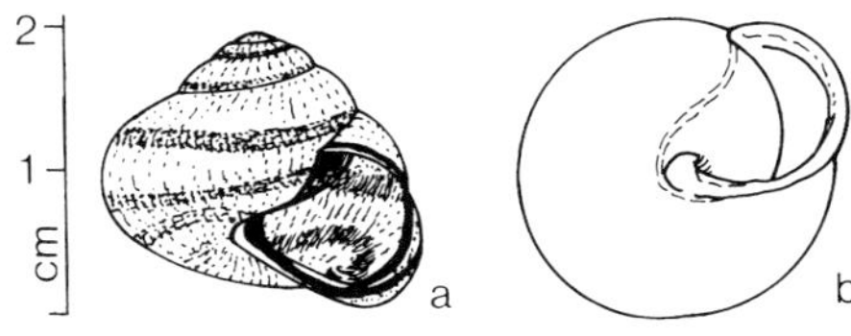
Fig. 9 Grove snail (*Cepaea moralis*). a) Lateral view, b) ventral view.

In captivity, development times are in our experience somewhat shorter. Both species reproduce after about a year if kept at a temperature of 19-23°C and allowed to hibernate for 4-5 months. Their life expectancy is about 3 years.

Container, Substrate, and Equipment: Suitable containers are a box like the one shown in Fig. 13, larger plastic tubs, or a variety of glass tanks that are covered with a tight screen top. A container of 50 x 40 x 40 cm can house 200 snails of varying sizes, not counting breeding stock. Wooden boxes are only suitable if they have been water-proved because of the high humidity requirements.

Suitable substrates consist of pulled-apart moss and unfertilized peat moss, or loose garden or forest soil, or a mixture of all of these. The substrate is filled into the container to about 10 cm height; depending on the number of inhabitants, it must be replaced every 4-8 weeks. The animals like to climb on branches.

When the weather is favorable, the setups can be placed outdoors in a protected area, otherwise indoors or in the basement. An incandescent light bulb provides light and gentle heat.

Food: Snails eat leaves of all kinds—they like burning nettles in particular—of rotting plants, alder flowers, and fruit. They also eat just about everything that is cultivated in a garden: lettuce, spinach, beans, carrots, potatoes, cucumbers, tomatoes, rutabaga, and sweet fruit. Old bran bread, soy flour, and water mixed together are a favorite power food. They will also eat the calcium off cuttlefish bones for building their shells.

Snails are rather susceptible to digestive problems when they eat feces and rotting or spoiled food. They need fresh food every couple of days; leftovers and feces must be removed carefully. Since the snails are active at night, they should be fed in the evening.

Breeding Conduitions:

Light: Snails are active at night, but they require a day-night rhythm to behave normally.

Temperature: The preferred temperature is 19-20°C. During the day it should rise to 23-24°C, and drop again at night. Hibernation is mandatory for breeding animals; they rest for 4-5 months at a temperature of 2-5°C.

Humidity: Everybody has most likely observed that snails are very active after a rainfall. Especially during the mating season they should be misted with luke-warm water every evening so that the humidity rises to 80-90%. The substrate should also be kept moist, but not muddy.

Notes: Much experience is still to be gained about breeding snails. It often appears that native animals are harder to keep and breed than tropical ones. The authors do not know of any large-scale snail breeders.

Spring is the best time to start breeding snails in order to get as many offspring as possible as soon as possible. The desired number of snails is collected toward the end of March; 30 snails should produce about 1000 offspring. The snails are placed in their prepared containers. They must be fed well on a varied diet, and feces and leftover food must be removed regularly. If you get lucky, you will witness courtship and mating. About 6-8 weeks after capture, the snails have usually deposited their first clutches of eggs. At the latest when these eggs hatch, the adults

should be moved to a new container.
During the first 3-4 weeks the shells of the
young snails are very soft and can be
crushed by their parents, or they are simply
eaten by them.

After the adults have laid their last eggs
around the middle of July, you can
try to coax them into a short early hibernation cycle to encourage them to produce
more eggs in the same year. Feed the
animals especially well in the last 2 weeks,
then put them into a wooden box filled
with moist moss to about 10 cm height.
Keep the animals warm, but do not
mist or feed anymore. After about a
week, the snails have retreated into their
shells and sealed them with a cover of
calcium that protects from dryness
and cold. After that, the snails can be
placed into a cotton bag, which in turn is
put into a small wooden box. After
about 3 weeks, this box is placed into the
refrigerator nightly at a temperature
of about 9°C; during the day, it is kept
in the coolest place in the house.
Thereafter, the snails remain in the
refrigerator for about 6 weeks at 2-4°C;
occasionally, the cotton bag should be
moistenedlightly.

By the beginning of October the snails are
reacquainted with warmer temperatures
in reverse order and by mid-November,
they are placed into a breeding container
and treated in the same way as newly
collected specimens. With a little luck, they
will produce another clutch of eggs by the
end of the year. However, this process
weakens the animals so much that only a
small percentage will survive a second
hibernation in March. So, at that point,
they are better used as food.

It must be considered whether it might be
better to just keep the snails in accordance
with their natural rhythm and have them
hibernate from October to the end of
February.

The offspring that is to be used as food can
be fed out during the winter. Some of the
snails can also be cooled down and
warmed up as needed. The strongest and
healthiest young specimens should be
selected in fall as breeding stock and
allowed th hibernate naturally. Some of
them will be ready to reproduce by the
following summer, some the following
spring.

Pests and Diseases: A single-celled
organism from the order of the
Coccidida, *Klossia helicina*, sometimes
occurs in the epithelium of the kidneys of
the snails. This parasite is harmless to the
snails and of no consequence to vivarium
animals. If kept under less than clean
conditions, the snails will easily develop
intestinal problems that will kill them
unless they are immediately moved to a
clean substrate.

Feeding: Most of the time the snails will
simply be placed into the terrarium or the
cage. To avoid unsightly slime tracks and
bite marks on plants, make sure they are
eaten soon. For small reptiles, the shell
should be crushed. The snails are killed
easily by boiling them in hot water
briefly. They can then be pulled out of their
shells and chopped up, for example to
feed cichlids.

Compared to the number of insect-eating
vivarium animals, the number that accepts
snails is comparatively modest. They
include colored sub-family Dipsadinae,
pink-tongued skinks (*Tiliqua gerrardii*),
and the Caiman lizard (*Dracaena
guianensis*). The latter two also accept a

small percentage of other foods. Tortoises, *Terrapene*-species and many lizards, like legless lizards, fence lizards, tegus, monitor lizards, and chameleons like snails as a supplemental food. Many birds and ground beetles (*Carabus auratus*) like snails quite a bit.

Advantages and Disadvantages:

Advantages:
- Excellent source of food
- Odor-free when kept properly
- Does not require high temperatures

Disadvantages:
- Large breeding containers
- Labor intensive
- Medium rate of reproduction and long development time

Giant African Land Snail (*Achatina fulica*)

NOTE BY TRANSLATOR: *These snails are illegal in the United States. If caught with them, you could be subject to a $5000 fine and up to 5 years in jail.*
In the early 70's a young boy, from Hawaii, was visiting his grandmother in the Miami area of Florida, and brought a few with him (from Hawaii). She decided to let them go in her back yard and they soon became a major agricultural pest, destroying entire orange groves. It took the US millions of dollars and several years to eliminate the pest from the state. They were introduced to California around the same time, presumably on a shipment form a foreign port. There too, they have been eliminated.
On Hawaii, they have literally taken over. They have forced several native species into extinction by eating all available food supplies. A carnivorous snail was imported from Africa, to destroy the Achatina fulica, but this turned out to be a worse problem. The carnivorous snail follows the trail of other snail and then eats them... the only problem was... they only eat snails that are smaller than them selves. Being only a fraction the size of A. fulica, they never ate any. They did, however start eating the remaining native snails. However, these snails are popular in Europe as food animals and sometimes pets.
It may be better not to include this chapter in the US Edition.

Description: The shell of the giant African land snail reaches a considerable size: up to 12 cm tall and 5 cm wide with a shiny yellowish to reddish brown mottled pattern. The lip is reddish and the body light to yellowish brown, about 18 cm long and 4.5 cm wide. The 1 cm long head has 2 pairs of tentacles, the 3.4 cm long eyestalks, and the 1.6 cm long front tentacles. The spherical or oval, thin-shelled, light-green eggs have a diameter of 5.5-6.0 mm. The hatchlings carry a shell that is 7 mm high and 6 mm wide.

Achatina fulica (Fig. 11), like all Achatinas originated in Africa. They were introduced into Asia and America and caused significant damage in agriculture.

Development Cycle: This snail prefers a daytime temperature between 25-26°C, and a nighttime temperature of 21-23°C. At these tem-peratures the eggs hatch in 14-18 days. The hatchlings grow amazingly fast: after 4 days the shell is 9 mm

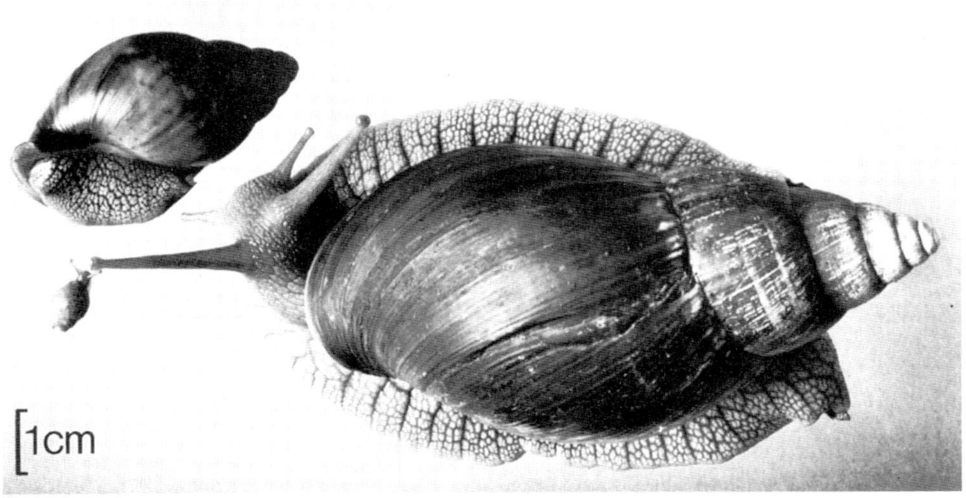

Fig. 11 Giant African land snail (*Achatina fulica*).

long by 7.5 mm wide and the animal weighs 70 mg; after 9 days the values are 12 x 9 mm and 1.6 g; after 14 days 15 x 13 mm and 2.45 g; after 4-5 weeks 31 x 21 mm and 5.6 g; after 7-9 weeks 37 x 24 mm and 8 g; after 12-13 weeks 46 x 26 mm and 15-17 g; after 6-7 months 80 x 36 mm and 40–44 g; after 13-14 months (adult snails) 120 mm x 50 mm and 90-100 g.

Being a tropical snail, *Achatina fulica* can reproduce year-round. The animals usually go through one rest period each year, which tends to fall in the winter months. They lay 30-90 eggs every 3-4 months into the ground, into cracks, or above ground. If the population density is high, the eggs are often dug up again; if they do not dry out, they will hatch anyway. *Achatina fulica* lives for a long time; it can reach an age of 10 years.

Containers, Substrate, and Equipment: The breeding container (Fig. 12) must be waterproof, therefore wooden boxes are

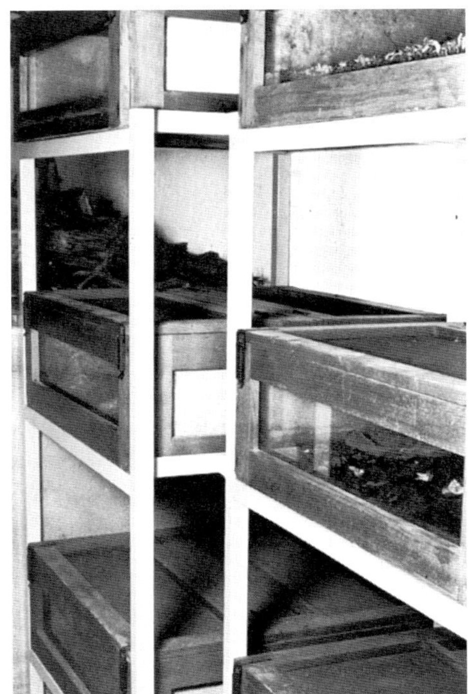

Fig. 12 Breeding setup for *Achatina fulica*.

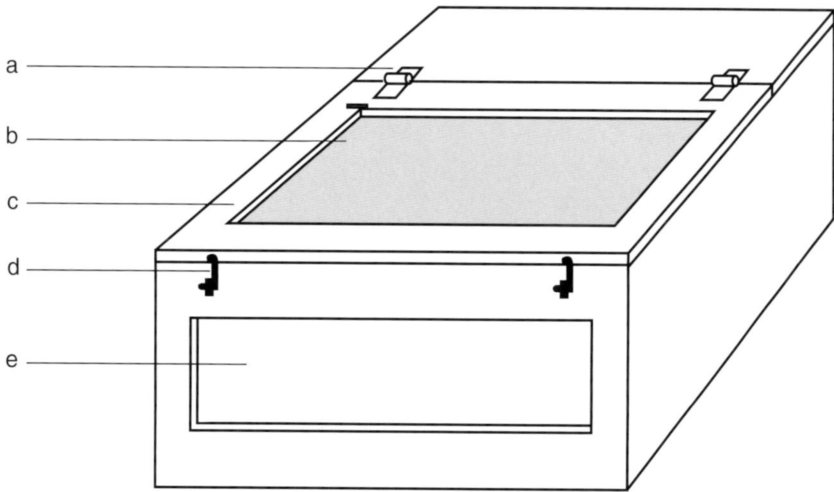

Fig. 13 Breeding container for *Achatina fulica* and snails home-made from coated wood or plastic. a) Hinge, b) mesh, c) cover, d) latch, e) glass pane.

only suitable if they are lined with plastic. Larger tanks on racks, plastic tubs, or a box as shown in Fig. 13 can be used. The lid must have a large mesh section.

The size of the animals requires large containers. For a small setup with 5 adult breeders and their offspring 1200-1500 cm^2 are appropriate, for example, 45 x 30 cm. On a surface of 60 x 50 cm up to 8 adult snails or 2000 juveniles of various sizes can be kept. The minimum height for the container is 30 cm.

Although it has not been observed that these snails can squeeze open the lid of their containers, the animals can show surprising strength and the lid should be secured with a latch.

Juvenile snails can also be kept in plastic baskets without a substrate until they reach sexual maturity. These baskets, whose holes should be just big enough for the feces to fall through, are suspended inside tubs. The required air humidity is reached by keeping them in a climate-controlled cabinet or by adding heated water to the tub. About 1-2 times a week the basked is rinsed with warm water and the tub cleaned. The breeding container is filled to 15 cm with moist, unfertilized peat moss and green moss, and furnished with a few pieces of bark for hiding places.

During the day, the snails like to bury themselves and hide while at night they wander around looking for food.

Ideally, the container is placed in a temperature-controlled room or cabinet. *Achatina fulica* do not like radiant heat, so the cabinet should not be heated with an infrared heat emitter but by 1-2 in candescent bulbs that are mounted outside the tub to prevent burns. Weak heat tape or heating pads are well suited, but for even heating and fire safety should be installed in a false bottom or underneath the container, and must not raise the tempera-ture above 26°C.

Food: *Achatina fulica* will eat any greens, vegetables, fruit that can be found, especially head lettuce, cucumbers, zucchinis, squash, raw potatoes, and rutabagas. Fruit and vegetables are cut in half and placed face-down in a small bowl. These snails are ravenous feeders: 20 adults can devour a whole head of lettuce or a 1/3-pound cucumber in one night. The snails require fresh food every other day. Leftovers must be carefully removed. The snails require constant access to calcium for building their shells. Bird grit, cuttlefish bone or a calcium block for birds or rodents should be provided. Lack of calcium will result in thin and fragile shells.

Breeding Conditions:

Light: A day-night cycle stimulates reproduction and is necessary. Moderate light during the day suffices.

Temperature: As mentioned, the optimal daytime temperature is at 25-26°C and 21-23°C for the night. This is also the narrow temperature range in which the snails eat well and breed. At 27-28°C they will withdraw and construct a lid even if the humidity is high. In this way they survive temperatures to 35°C, but none below 15°C.

Humidity: The snails will only eat and breed if the substrate and air humidity are high. Air humidity should be 70-90%. If the snails are kept too dry, they will withdraw and construct a lid; they can rest for up to half a year in that manner.

Notes: The only known breeding setups are of small or medium scale, except when these snails are bred as a delicacy for human consumption.

With 5-15 adult snails, a breeding setup can be made that delivers about 750-2200 food snails.

If only two animals are kept, no offspring may result because the animals lay infertile eggs. Could it be because the two animals are not ready to mate at the same time? However, in larger groups specimens can also be found that will not produce eggs for a whole year.

The daily chores include spraying, feeding, and removing feces and food leftovers; the best time to take care of the animals is in the evening, before they become active. The substrate is watered once a week and replaced every 2-8 weeks, depending on population density. Snails easily get digestive problems if the substrate is dirty or if they eat rotten food.

A medium-sized breeding setup with 20-40 breeders can still fit into a cabinet of the appropriate size. However, it is better to use two containers: Newly hatched snails and eggs that are found are moved to a second container, or the young snails are raised in baskets.

If no snails are needed for a longer period, a vacation is inevitable, the snails can be put into estivation. The spraying, watering and feeding is halted, and barely a week later the animals will have closed up their shells. (Snails only construct lids when their intestines are empty.) They tolerate estivation for up to six months. They are stored at room temperature, which must not fall below 15°C.

To reawaken the snails they are sprayed daily and the temperature is raised. After a few days, their lids come off and they start to feed again. Courtship behaviors start two weeks later and offspring can be expected, which is especially numerous after a resting period. These snails can go without food for 2-3 weeks without damage if they have been fed well beforehand. If they are kept moist, they will simply bury themselves in the substrate without closing up.

Pests and Diseases: No significant parasites are known for *Achatina fulica*. If kept clean, digestive problems can be avoided. Springtails are often introduced with dirt or food, but they have no negative effect on the setup.

Feeding: *Achatina fulica* grows so large that adult animals can only be fed to monitor lizards. However, when they are the size of hazelnuts or walnuts they make perfect food items for the same animals as described for the garden and grove snails. It is also described there how to offer them.

Advantages and Disadvantages:

Advantages:
- Excellent source of food
- Large range of size of animals
- Odor free when kept clean
- Survive several months in estivation

Disadvantages:
- Breeding requires a lot of space
- High cost of food
- Labor intensive

Crustaceans

The crustaceans are with 35,000 species not just a large but also a varied class of animals. Most crustaceans live in the ocean, many in freshwater, quite a few as parasites, and only a small number on land. Inhabitants of all areas, parasites excluded of course, provide us with necessary food animals. In the following sections the breeding of water fleas, brine shrimp, and pillbugs is described. Daphniae and *Moina* (family Daphniidae) belong to the suborder of water fleas (Cladocera) and belong together with *Artemia salina* (family Branchinectidae in the order Anostraca) to the subclass of the Branchiopoda. The isopods (order Isopoda) belong to the higher crustaceans of the subclass Malacostraca. Representatives of three families are discussed: Oniscidae with *Oniscus*, Porcellionidae with *Porcellio*, and Armadillidiidae with *Armadillidium*.

To better understand the listed species the shape and forms of crustaceans are briefly discussed. Crustaceans, like insect arthropods have bodies protected by an external chitin skeleton, which is often fortified by calcium deposits. Their bodies are divided into several segments that can be summarized as the head, thorax, and abdomen. However, the number of segments is not as fixed as for the insects. Often one or more thoracic segments are fused with the head to form a celaphothorax, the remaining segments forming a middle body called the pereon, and the abdomen. The isopods do have a thoracic segment that is fused with their head.

Basically, each segment has one pair of appendages (exopods) that are adapted to a variety of uses, for example the antennae, the mouthparts, or the walking legs. The thoracic exopods are generally used for propulsion and have some kind of gills in water-dwelling crustaceans. The daphniae, however, have a second antenna that has been rebuilt into a strong rowing appendage, and the thoracic legs are primarily used to move food towards the month. The abdomen of water fleas and brine shrimp has no exopods; in the isopods they are

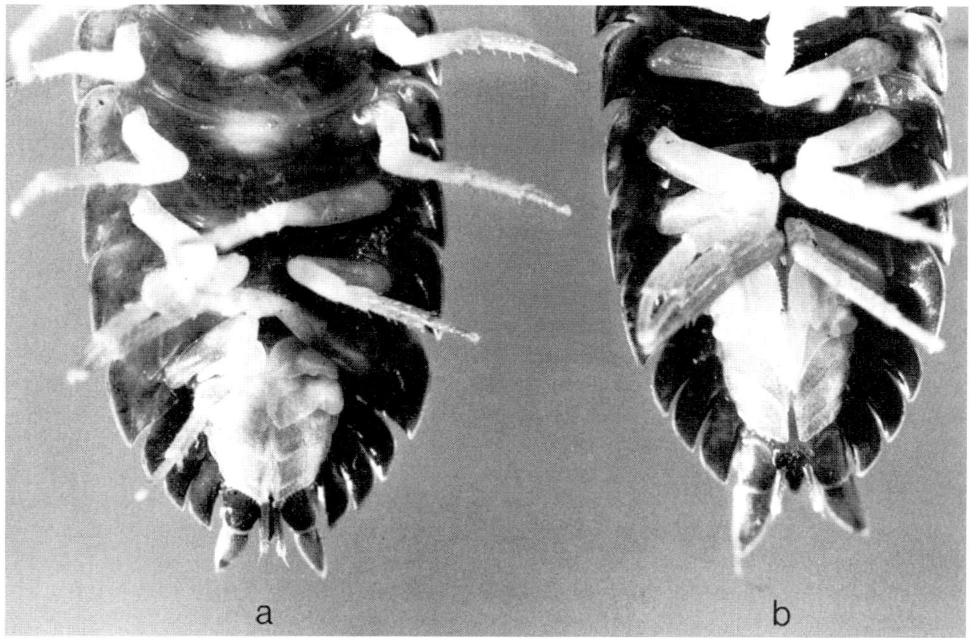

Fig. 14   Underside of *Oniscus asellus*. a) Pregnant female, b) male.

adapted as a breathing apparatus. In addition, a part of the second and often the first abdominal exopods form an organ that the isopod males use during mating; this makes it easy to determine their gender with the naked eye (Fig. 14).

Water fleas have a kind of shell that starts behind their head and covers their whole body like a mantle. This shell consists, like the skin, of more or less calcified chitin. Crustaceans usually lay fertilized eggs from which larvae hatch that grow after several molts into adult animals. Several types of larvae are known and given different designations.

The nauplius larvae are worth mentioning; they are a simple form of larva that consists of only three segments. On the other hand, daphniae and terrestrial isopods, for example, hatch as complete little crustaceans that only need to grow to adult size. For some crustaceans, the eggs hatch inside the female's body, and even unfertilized eggs can develop (parthenogenesis). It is noteworthy that terrestrial isopod females deposit their eggs into a special brooding pouch, which consists of five oostegites that grow from the inside of the hip of the first five thoracic extremities, form a leaf shape, and overlap in the middle of the underside. The brooding pouch closes tightly and is filled with liquid, so that the embryos develop in a miniature pond until they hatch. This makes the terrestrial isopods completely independent of water. The oostegites form during one of the molts called the parturial ecdysis.

Large Water Flea
(*Daphnia magna*)
Water Flea
(*Daphnia pulex*)
Russian Daphnia
(*Moina macrocopa*)

Who is not familiar with them? And who of the older generations has not ventured out to catch some? Their name derives from their jumping way of swimming. In accordance with their genus *Daphnia* they are commonly and collectively called daphniae or water fleas. There are several hundred species, but only a few have gained significance as fish food. Usually they are representatives of *Daphnia magna* and *Daphnia pulex* (Fig. 15). Another daphnia has been introduced to Europe from Japan, but it has disappeared again even though it is easy to breed. *Moina macrocopa* lives in ponds that dry out for part of the year; this explains their tolerance for poor water quality.

Description: The whole body is covered by a shell-like carapace and the rostrum is pointed and powerful. The quite complex eyes have grown together and can be clearly seen on the head in addition to the first pair of small antennae, which are covered with sensory organs. The second pair of antennae are large, forked, and covered with bristles that are used for swimming; this is how the daphnia moves: it beats the antennae and thus jumps forward. The thoracic segments have five pairs of leaf-like legs. Water fleas have a paired claw (furca) at the tail end of the legless abdomen. It is used to remove unwanted particles from underneath the

50

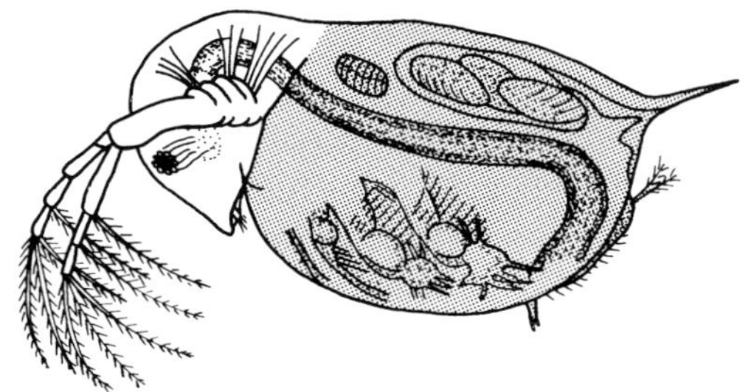

Fig. 15 Common water flea (*Daphnia pulex*).

carapace. The legs are used to filter food but also have gills. Under the microscope the heartbeat can be observed in these transparent crustaceans, as well as the eggs and the unborn young in the brooding pouch of the females. The two *Daphnia* species reach a size of 6 mm, while *Moina* reaches 1.8-2 mm. Under ideal living conditions, daphnia show an intense red coloring.

Development Cycle: Daphniae can be found in any pond that offers some nutrients, and they occur in masses in ponds where ducks and other waterfowl live, be it in zoos, or, less often, in town ponds. The bird droppings fertilize the water, and algae and single-celled organisms grow in large quantities. They are the primary source of food for daphniae who filter-feed on them.

In spring, primarily females that multiply through parthenogenesis are found. At high temperatures, their development is very fast. Young females reach sexual maturity within a few days, which leads to observable population explosions. In theory, one female can produce several million offspring in one summer. Males appear later in the year. They mate with the females, which then produce eggs that survive through the cold time of the year.

Waterfowl disperse them between different bodies of water.

Catching and Keeping Daphnia: Once an unpolluted body of water has been located, a fine-meshed net, a bucket, or even better, a frame covered with gauze, fabric, or fine wire-mesh can be used to acquire daphnia. The net is pulled through the water in a figure-eight pattern. The catch is dropped into a bucket (not too many since daphniae require a lot of oxygen!) or spread on the frame in a thin layer which is covered with wet newspaper or cloth. At home, everything is dumped into a container, which because of the chlorine content should not be filled with fresh tap water but only with water that has been left standing for a few days. After the dead animals have settled, siphon the food animals with a hose into a sieve. This pretty much prevents the introduction of uninvited guests and the food is pretty clean.

To keep some of the animals, live ones are transferred into a large container that must not be made of metal, in shallow water, and placed in a cool spot. If there are many animals, aeration is useful. The daphniae should not be subject to temperature shock during transfer. In this manner, they should keep for a few days even in summer.

Breeding Daphnia: If large tubs made of concrete or plastic, or old barrels, can be set up outdoors in a sunny location, breeding can be attempted. The water can be as shallow as 50 cm, but the surface area should be as large as possible. First, the water is seeded with organic substances to grow food. Baking yeast, milk, egg powder, or small pieces of meat can be soaked in water for a while and the resulting "broth" can be added to the tubs. Only add small amounts and dose according to the amount of water in the containers. After a few days, enough organisms should have grown, and if the containers are in the sun, there should also be algae. Now the daphniae can be added. In a short while, they will filter the murky water back to clear. If careful feeding continues, they will multiply rapidly. The same method can be used for a small natural pond. However, such a pond should be free of fish and have as few other inhabitants as possible. Excess daphniae can be frozen for winter and thawed later to make an excellent food. Frozen daphniae can also be bought from aquarium stores.

If a cool room that is protected from winter frost is available, the daphnia breeding setup can be moved there for the cold season. If fed well but carefully, they breed even in winter. Of course, every so often, at least a partial water change will be necessary, and feces, skins, and dead animals should be siphoned off from time to time.

Container for *Moina macrocopa*: This undemanding crustacean can be bred in containers of less than a gallon. Large pickling jars or small aquariums work well They are filled with tap water that has stood for at least 24 hours at about 22°C and set up in a bright spot out of direct sunlight. To prevent a film from forming at the surface, gentle aeration is recommended.

Food and Hints for Breeding *Moina macrocopa*: Another advantage of these animals is that they can be fed with yeast that has been started in a bowl of warm water. If feedings start slowly, and are then increased, the water fleas will multiply rapidly and food animals can be harvested after about 8 days. The best amount of food must be determined carefully by trial and error. The water should be clear about 24 hours after food has been added. Such a setup works for about 3 weeks, then it starts to smell and the red coloring of the water fleas fades.

This indicates that it is time to start a new setup. All the animals are filtered out and transferred into fresh water. It is advantageous to have several setups at different stages so that sufficient food animals are always available.

Breeding Conditions:

Light: Water fleas require light. If no natural light is available, artificial light must be substituted, preferably with a fluorescent light or possibly with an incandescent bulb.

Temperature: All water fleas breed well at a temperature of 20-25°C. If they are kept outdoors, the temperature can be higher; in winter, a lower temperature of 15-18°C is recommended, otherwise the crustaceans might die from lack of oxygen. *Moina* does best at a year-round temperature of 20-25°C.

Feeding: The water fleas are carefully siphoned off with a hose, strained, and perhaps rinsed with lukewarm water since they do not tolerate harsh changes in temperatures. The *Moina* is a lot more robust in that respect and tolerates rapid changes in temperature. Since daphnia use a lot of oxygen, not too many should be put into the aquarium. Uneaten or dead animals must be removed so that they will not spoil the water.

Daphnia are an excellent food for freshwater fish but can also be used for many tropical marine fish, for cichlids, angelfish, boxfish, puffer fish, sterlets, and bichirs. They can also be fed in lieu of plankton to seahorses and sea feathers.

Daphnia are useful for raising water turtles. In addition, salamander larvae will eat them. The carotene in the water fleas helps colored species form and maintain their yellow and red coloring. For example, when daphnia are fed to flamingos in large quantities, they maintain their pink color; they are also a natural food for these birds.

Advantages and Disadvantages:

Advantages:
* If done right, straightforward
* Possible to keep outdoors (summer only)
* Excellent food
* Large yield

Disadvantages:
* Requires large amounts of space, except *Moina*
* Possibility of introducing parasites and pests into the aquariums, especially when caught wild

Brine Shrimp
(*Artemia salina*)

More appropriately, the title should be "*Artemia gracilis*, the American brine shrimp," since most commercially available brine shrimp eggs originate from salt lakes in the United States. Their skin is impermeable to salt, which allows them to survive in this extreme environment with changing salt concentration. Salt that is taken in with food is excreted through special appendages on their legs.

Description: Fully-grown brine shrimp are 12-15 mm long. The 15 body segments have 11 pairs of legs that are used for swimming and filter feeding (on small detritus). The color of the shrimp varies from pink to bright red depending on the salt concentration. The males have pincer-shaped antennae, while the females have visible egg sacks behind their swimming legs. The animals swim almost constantly and with belly-up.

When bodies of water dry out, the salt concentration increases. The brine shrimp deposit so-called cysts of about 0.2 mm diameter, in which embryo development comes to a halt after a few cell divisions (diapause). These "eggs" can be bought at aquarium stores. Stored dry, they remain viable for years.

The nauplius larvae are drop-shaped, about 0.5 mm long, with strong antennae that are used for swimming. If the salt concentration is low, the larvae hatch in the females' body shortly before deposition. If the nauplius larvae find enough food, they molt in short intervals. Their shape stretches out, and the swimming legs develop, which are now used for propulsion. The animals are sexually mature—that is, they are not larvae anymore—after the 17th molt.

Development Cycles and Temperature Requirements: Once the eggs are put into saltwater, they hatch within 1-3 days depending on the temperature. At 15-20°C after 48 hours, at 24°C after 24-36 hours. Brine shrimp tolerate variations in temperature well. Newly hatched nauplius larvae can be refrigerated at 4°C for up to a week. At room temperature, they would die within 3 days. For a high-yield breeding setup, consistently higher temperatures are required. It makes sense to heat the tub or aquarium with heat tape or a submersible aquarium heater.

At 20°C, the brine shrimp reach sexual maturity in 37 days, at 30°C already in 18 days. At an optimal feeding rate of around the clock they can be fully grown in 18-21 days at 20°C, and in 12 days at 28°C. The hobbyist is unlikely to accomplish this, however. Unfortunately, no data are available on lifespan or reproduction rate.

Light Requirements: For cultures where the nauplius larvae are simply hatched and then used as food, no special lighting is required. If the animals are grown to sexual maturity, a strong source of light is required so that green algae can grow. This keeps the water clear, and the algae, once they are scraped of the sides of the containers and float free, make a good supplementary food for the nauplius larvae. If no location with natural sunlight is available, a light source can be installed above the container; it should be left on for 12 hours ever day.

Breeding Containers and Notes on Small Setups: Since the price for brine shrimp eggs has been rising, breeding them has gained significance even for the hobbyist. The simplest ways are shown here with hints toward the more elaborate setup options. For most aquarium enthusiasts, who only keep a few tanks for their enjoyment, the investment into a larger breeding setup is not worth the trouble. Often there will not be enough time to take care of a labor-intensive breeding setup. For the hobbyist, commercially available brine shrimp hatchery kits are excellent, even though the yield is moderate: this can be done by using the "bottle method" or the "incubator method." This relatively cheap equipment is sufficient for most daily needs.

Another option is to breed in large, shallow containers, for example, those used to develop photographs, that can be placed on a porch or balcony in summer. They are filled with saltwater to 6-7 cm and placed in the sun. As soon as the pan shows good algae growth, eggs or freshly hatched nauplius larvae are added. The algae are the best food and the animals will grow fast. Evaporated water is replaced. Once the nauplius larvae have consumed all the algae, they must be fed as described in the section on "Feeding." Large glass tanks or plastic tubs of 15-18 cm height can also be used for breeding. The amount of time for upkeep can be reduced by creating relatively natural conditions. For this, the bottom is covered with a 3-5 cm layer of garden soil and then filled with about 10 cm of ocean water (Siepe, 1977). About 100 nauplius larvae are added for each liter of water. The soil contains many microorganisms, and single-celled animals develop continually, which serve as food for the nauplius larvae. In this setup, supplemental feeding is only needed after 2-3 weeks. Adult brine shrimp disturb the bottom in their search for food, so feedings must proceed carefully even when the water is murky. For all setups, it must be kept in mind that at the high temperatures of 25-30° C, the oxygen content of the water is reduced and aeration is especially important. It also influences the hatch rate, as more hatchlings can be freed of their egg shells if the water is moving. Aeration should, however, not be so strong that the bottom or the animals are moved around.

Finally, a very simple method of hatching must be mentioned; one that is especially suitable for those who have little space available. Fill a petri or other shallow dish with saltwater to a height of about 2 cm. Since the water is shallow, no aeration is required. Put a feeding ring (like the ones most aquarium hobbyists own) in the section of the dish that faces away from the light. Sprinkle eggs into the feeding ring; the egg shells will later remain in the ring. If possible, the light should be directed so that the nauplius larvae will congregate in the brightest area. In that way they can be removed with a pipette.

Cultivation Medium: One of the most important factors when breeding brine shrimp is the salt. If the eggs are only kept until they hatch, it does not matter whether sea salt or table salt is used; only iodized salt is not suitable. However, to raise and breed brine shrimp sea salt is preferred; recommended is a premixed salt mixture for breeding brine shrimp, which can be purchased. Those mixtures were developed especially for brine shrimp, and it is not necessary to mix one's own.

However, if you make your own ocean water, a density of $1024 g/cm^3$ is good for breeding brine shrimp. At 20°C this is equivalent to a concentration of 3.4%; that is, about 34 g of salt must be dissolved in 1 l of water. Water from a saltwater fishtank can also be used after it has been filtered clean. Brine shrimp can be successfully bred in water that has a salt content between 1.5-4%; that is, a density between 1.0097-1.0286 g/cm^3 at 20°C. The lower concentrations allow bacteria to develop more easily.

The water density can be determined with an areometer. It is acceptable to use hard tap water since the water's calcium content is not relevant. It is beneficial to let the saltwater stand for a few days and possibly aerate it before using it. Since evaporation increases the salt concentration, the water must then be topped off with freshwater (that has also been left standing).

Brine shrimp are rather tolerant of variations in the salt concentration; they are also not very sensitive to waste products that accumulate in the water.

After running the setup for a while, it is recommended to change 1/3 of the water.

Food: The easiest food for brine shrimp is yeast. In setups that use garden soil as their bottom substrate, it has proven excellent. Fresh (live) yeast cubes can be bought in various places (e.g., health food stores). Put the yeast in a bowl with a little bit of warm water and stir carefully until the whole cube has mostly dissolved.

Let the bowl sit for a while. Yeast that has been prepared in this way will keep for weeks in the refrigerator. Dry fish food, especially TetraPhyll, alone or mixed with TetraMin, also brings good results according to Zahn (1972). It is important that the dry food be pulverized with a mortar and pestle and then mixed with water until it forms a homogeneous paste; brine shrimp can only eat the smallest particles. Depending on the size of the setup and its population density, food is offered daily in amounts ranging from a few drops to several milliliters of the yeast or dry food preparation. Some authors recommend a dust-like powder made from grinding up stinging nettles or algae. Alternatively, a commercial brine shrimp food can be purchased, which consists of salts, trace elements, and phytoplankton.

Another excellent and natural food for brine shrimp are freshwater plankton (see section on breeding plankton). A container, preferably made from glass or Plexiglas, is inoculated with a little bit of phytoplankton and placed in a bright location, but not in direct sunlight. After a while, the plankton has multiplied and the water is intensely green. To feed the brine shrimp, enough of the liquid to color the water light green is poured into the brine shrimp tank. Careful! The freshwater plankton dies fast in the saltwater. After a while, the water becomes clear again.

If you have a breeding setup for *Dunaliella* (see section on saltwater plankton), you have of course no problems feeding your brine shrimp.

The success of a brine shrimp breeding setup depends significantly on feeding the right amounts of food; deciding on how much that is can be tricky. Nauplius larvae and the adult shrimp are ravenous eaters. However, they should only be fed as much as they can eat it up in 12 hours. Otherwise, bacteria will develop and pollute the setup. More food should be added only after the water becomes completely clear again.

Only if *Dunaliella* are fed, more generous amounts of food can be offered.

Feeding: Catching brine shrimp is easy: Cover the container so that light only reaches it in one place. After a short time, the brine shrimp, who crave light, will congregate there. They can be siphoned off with a hose and strained through a fine-meshed sieve. After rinsing them with freshwater, they can then be fed to the vivarium animals.

Adult brine shrimp are an excellent food for all fish and lower animals, like anemones. Freshly hatched nauplius larvae make an excellent food for plankton eaters such as tubeworms, corals, young seahorses, and pipefish. Of course, they can also be used to raise freshwater and saltwater fish fry.

Large-scale Breeding: This topic shall only be touched on lightly. Of course, large fishtanks always require large amounts of food. In this case, it is worthwhile to breed brine shrimp in containers of 500 l. In such setups, electrical agitators keep the water in constant motion. At the same time, these gigantic agitators move waste products into especially designed depressions. Often, a timer-controlled pump provides feeding solution in measured amounts at specified intervals. Algae or fish food suspensions have been used as food with good results.

For more information on large-scale setups, refer to articles in specialist journals.

Advantages and Disadvantages:

Advantages:
- Eggs are commonly available
- Rich in nutrients and suitable even for sensitive animals
- Impossible to introduce pests into the breeding containers

Disadvantages:
- Large amount of work
- Setups must be checked twice daily
- Neglected or forgotten setups develop strong odor

56

Woodlouse
(*Oniscus asellus*)
Woodlouse
(*Porcellio scaber*)
Pillbug
(*Armadillidium nasatum*)
Pillbug
(*Armadillidium vulgare*)

Description: *Oniscus asellus* (Fig. 16): The body is wide-ovoloid and flat, 15-18 mm long, 6-10.5 mm wide, and 1.5-2 mm high, mostly shiny and black-brown to reddish brown in color with lighter patterns along both sides of the middle of the back. The lateral parts of the pereon segments extend flattened. The visible antennae consist of a basal peduncle of five articles and a distal, whiplike flagellum of three articles that is typically angled. The third article of the flagellum is about three times as long as the first one. On underside of the abdomen, there are no white spots.

At a length of about 7 mm and an age of four months, these animals are sexually mature. The number of eggs increases with increasing size of the female from 13 for the first clutch to up to 80 for fully grown animals. In average, a 12 mm female deposits 43 eggs. The hatching young measure about 2 mm. Life expectancy is 3-4 years.

Porcellio scaber (Fig. 16): This animal reaches about the same size as *Oniscus asellus* but is narrower and it lacks the flattened pereon segments. The predominant color is a dull dark gray, occasionally lighter around the edges; or sometimes uniformly light reddish, yellowish, or whitish patterned animals can be found.

The flagella of the antennae only have two articles. On the underside of the abdomen, on the first two segments, two white spots can be seen; these are the breathing tubes, which are highly developed air breathing organs. The females lay more eggs than *Oniscus asellus*, an average of 57 at a length of 12 mm, and up to 119 for 17 mm long females.

Armadillidium vulgare and *A. nasatum* (Fig. 17): The body is domed, up to 4 mm thick, and can be completely rolled into a ball. The animals reach a length of 21 mm and a width of 11 mm for (*A. vulgare*) and 7 mm for (*A. nasatum*), but usually they stay smaller. The dark gray to brownish males of *A. nasatum* usually lack a lighter stripe along the back and are darker than the females. Both genders have short white lines along the sides of their backs. The young and females of *A. vulgare* show a mottled pattern of light yellow or reddish on dark brown; the males appear single-colored dark to lead gray. Both species occasionally produce reddish, red, or albino animals. All of them have two pairs of breathing tubes.

The two species are easily distinguished by their heads: The noselike protrusion of *A. nasatum* is easily recognized with the naked eye. If the animals are inspected from the side, it can be noted that the first abdominal segment of *A. nasatum* is indented, while that of *A. vulgare* is only somewhat rounded. For the latter species, it is known that they can live up to four years old.

These animals, too, lay more eggs as they get larger. The number for *A. nasatum* is 14-200, and up to 300 (!). For *A. vulgare*, however, the newly hatched young of this

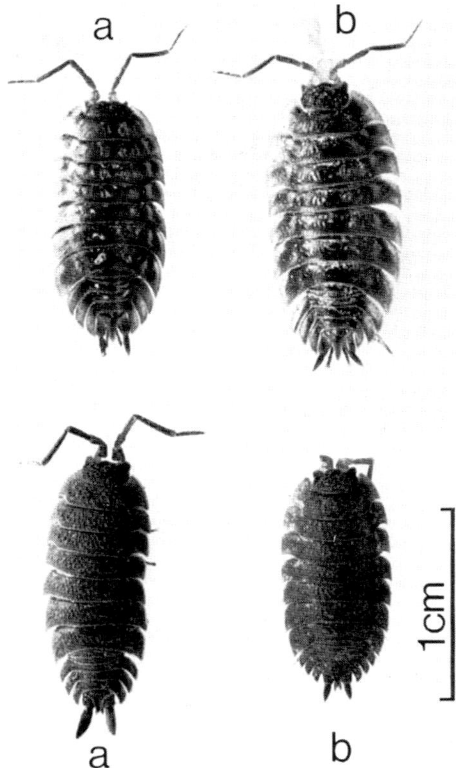

Fig. 16 Top: *Oniscus asellus*, bottom: *Porcellio scaber*. a) Male, b) female

species measure only 1.5 mm. With their soft, uncalcified skin (cuticle), they are as sensitive to drying out as *Oniscus asellus*.

All woodlice and pillbugs can be found easily near houses and gardens, under rocks, wood, and leaves. They can also be found in greenhouses. This is where *A. nasatus*, who likes it warm, can be found most frequently, while outdoors it can only be found in places that are protected from freezing in winter.

Development Times: As for all exotherms, development depends on the temperature.

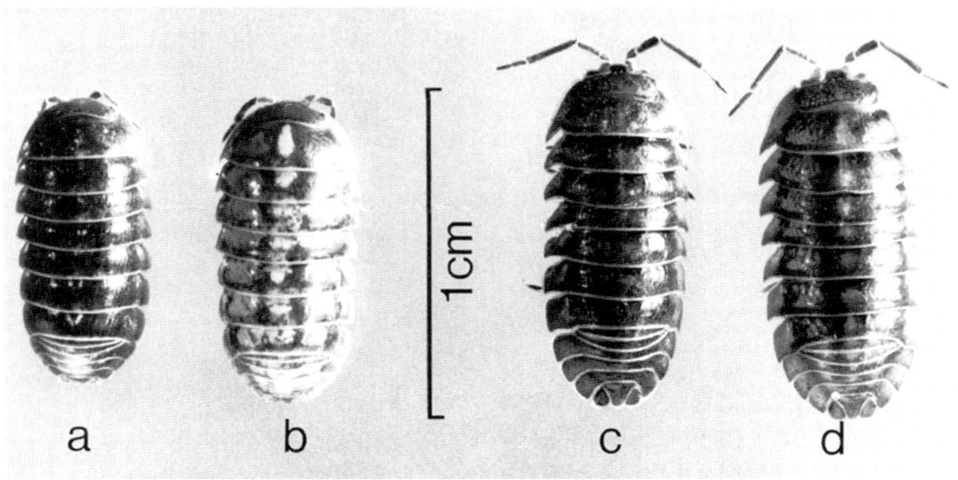

Fig. 17   a) and b) *Armadillidium vulgare*, c) and d) *Armadillidium nasatum*. a) and c) males, b) and d) females.

Best known are the development times for *A. vulgare*. The time from egg laying to hatching is 14 days at 30°C, 21 days at 25°C, 28 days at 22°C, 42-48 days at 18°C, and 70-77 days at 14°C. At lower temperatures, the embryos cannot develop. After five molts, the sex can be determined; at 30°C, this takes 28-35 days, at 18°C 63-70 days.

For *Oniscus asellus,* it is known that the embryos hatch after 47-49 days at 17-20°C. *Porcellio scaber* develops faster: at 20°C hatching occurs after an average of 27 days. Under good conditions, the next generation can hatch after only 6 weeks. The authors do not know of other data that have been collected under controlled conditions. They believe that each species can be induced to propagate every 8-12 weeks.

Containers, Substrate, Food, and Equipment: Any waterproof container with smooth sides of at least 20 cm height is suitable for breeding. Tubs, buckets, and old Plexiglas or glass tanks all work. For the woodlice, which love humidity, the container should be covered with a glass pane or a transparent plastic sheet that is not airtight. The animals cannot climb the straight sides, and they need air to breathe. The tub for the pillbugs, which tolerate more dryness, can remain open.

The lowest layer of the substrate consists of 2-4 cm of garden soil, which absorbs water well. On top of the soil, add 10-15 cm of moist leaf litter, which should be soft and partially decomposed and mixed with a few pieces of rotting wood that are covered with fungal growth. Directly on top of the leaf litter or on a pottery shard half of a slightly carved out potato or carrot is placed. Some old mortar, chalk, or powdered eggshell provides calcium. All this will be eaten over time. The animals eat primarily soft, decomposing plant matter, including fallen leaves, and small amounts of fresh plant matter like soaked seeds and seedlings, roots, and all sorts of vegetables like potatoes, carrots, black radishes, and fruit such as apples. They also eat fungus mycelium and animal matter; for example, they consume mites and eat dead, unpoisoned snails. A partially buried piece of wood and two flat rocks arranged on top of each other as a shelter complete the setup for the woodlice.

For the calcium-loving pillbugs, which prefer dryer surroundings, one half of the container is set up as follows: On top of the garden soil calcium-rich rocks are placed, and the leaves of the other half are mixed with fine rubble that is rich in calcium. For the woodlice the leaf layer is kept moist, not wet, at all times; for the pillbugs, the rocks are occasionally misted.

Breeding Conditions:

Light: Woodlice and pillbugs are active at night and only move around when it is light to find a new hiding place if the current one becomes too wet or too dry. However, it is wrong to think that these animals can be kept in a dark basement. They respond to light cycles, even when the light is very dim (50-100 lx). Under natural conditions, the females bear young three times in the course of a year, from spring to summer. If they are kept under artificial lighting for 16-hours each day, they breed last in fall and then again in March. If the cultures are switched to a shorter day (7 hours of light), it encourages them to breed, but a smaller percentage of the females than in the cultures with long days will breed (Wieser, 1963). These results are difficult to interpret. Our experience is that *Porcellio scaber* reproduces year-round in a room that receives light for several hours a day at irregular intervals.

Temperature: The following temperatures have been determined as preferred at a 100% relative humidity: *Oniscus asellus* female, 11-14°C, male, 15-18° C; *Porcellio scaber* female, 7-11°C, male, 12.5°C; *A. vulgare*, female, 14-19°C, and males 19-21°C. For *A. nasatum*, the values are probably slightly higher. For fast reproduction, higher temperatures are required, 18-20°C for the woodlice and 25°C for the pillbugs.

Humidity: As mentioned before, these animals require uniformly high humidity, but not wetness. Regular spraying of the leaf litter, preferably with a spray bottle, is necessary.

Notes: If the instructions in the previous sections are followed, the setup takes care of itself. It is better not to stir up the leaf litter, which can disturb molting animals. At least 30 females and 20 males are a good starting breeding stock. The animals should be left to reproduce for a few weeks to months before harvesting begins. For practical reasons, one might start breeding setups in summer and let them reproduce until winter while catching wild woodlice and pillbugs in the meantime.

The animals can be harvested in several ways. They can be selected from the animals that are hiding underneath the potato, wood, or rocks. By tapping on the hiding place, they will drop into a ready glass. Schöne (1979) suggests exploiting the fact that they cannot climb smooth walls. A smooth walled can whose outer surface is roughened (cover with glue and sprinkle with sand) is placed into the breeding container. The animals climb the outside, fall into the can, and can be sorted at leisure. Daily control is important to prevent dehydration of the captives. The can should be removed or food added to it if it cannot be emptied for some days.

Pests and Diseases: No diseases are known to us. Wolf spiders, which can be introduced with the leaves, should not be tolerated because they like to eat woodlice and pillbugs. Springtails, which are also brought in the soil and the leaf litter should not affect the setup.

Feeding: Not all animals will eat woodlice or pillbugs, but some absolutely love them. This means trying it out and repeated offering. Some saltwater fish love them, for example blennies (Blenniidae) and porcupine fish (Teraodontidae) (according to Quitschau, 1976, and Schöne, 1979). For toads and terrestrial salamanders they are welcome treats, and many lizards, especially chameleons, and water turtles like them for variety. Wolf spiders, funnel-web spiders, solpugids, bird spiders, and scorpions also eat woodlice and pillbugs.

Advantages and Disadvantages:

Advantages:

- Woodlice and pillbugs require little upkeep
- Breeding is without risks as escaped animals dehydrate and die
- Especially suitable for nocturnal vivarium animals like frogs, toads, and geckos

Disadvantages:

- Only moderately productive
- Birds do not like them, especially not pillbugs

Insects

The number of insects, also called Hexapoda, is myriad and impossible to grasp. With over 100,000 species they are not only the largest class of animals, but in sheer number of species they surpass all the other groups taken together. Furthermore, it is amazing that they all share the same segmentation of the body and the same number of legs. Head, chest (thorax), and back (abdomen) can always be distinguished. The head has eyes, antennae, and mouthparts that allow them to consume different kinds of foods depending on their structure. The thorax consists of three segments that are rigidly connected and each segment has one pair of legs. The two posterior segments usually have a pair of wings each, leaf-like skin flaps that give insects a significant

ability: flight. Only archaic insects, which include the springtails, do not have wings. The flexible abdomen, which consists of a maximum of 11 segments (6 for springtails), never has legs in adult insects.

All insects lay eggs. Further development falls into two main categories: those insects that go through incomplete metamorphosis (hemimetabolous insects) and those who go through complete metamorphosis (holometabolous insects). In the first group, small larvae that look very similar to adults hatch from the eggs. After several molts, usually 5-8, they are mature and stop molting. Only after molting to the adult state, the imago, are they sexually mature, and the wings, which were only present as wing buds, unfold fully. Cockroaches, crickets, grasshoppers, and also springtails belong to this group. For the latter the adult animals can only be distinguished from the juvenile because their genitals are functional after a certain molt and the animals become sexually active. Adult springtails will still molt several times.

For insects with complete metamorphosis, a larva that has no similarity to the finished insect hatches from the egg and often has its own name, like "caterpillar" or "maggot." This mobile and ravenous larva transforms into an immobile, resting pupa. During the pupa stage, the animal changes profoundly and becomes the imago, which emerges from the pupa after a time. This group includes beetles, flies, and butterflies.

Springtails (Collembola)

The springtails form their own order (Collembola). These small, archaic insects with a body size of 0.2-9 mm are represented worldwide with over 3500 species. They live in a wide range of environments, for example, coastal areas, caves, bird nests, and even snow and ice on mountains or lake surfaces, where they can appear in enormous numbers. Springtails that live in straw or the upper layers of soil help decompose leaves and other plant matter. They are important members of the chain of organisms that convert
soil to humus. Their common name refers to the remarkable way in which they move. The "tail" is actually a paired appendage of the fourth abdominal segment, the so-called "furcula." When at rest, the furcula is folded under and held underneath the body; it is held in place with a clasp-like structure of the third segment, the tenaculum. To jump, the animal uses strong muscle action to pull the furcula out of the tenaculum and catapult itself up and forward, almost like a

toy jumping frog. A few species have furculas that are so strongly developed that they can jump 20 cm and further. Those species that live in the ground have no furcula. There are many intermediate types between those extremes.

Another organ that is unique to Collembolas is the ventral tube on the first abdominal segment to which research has attributed a variety of tasks: to help hold on to surfaces, to right the animal after a jump, to take in water and help gill breathing, as well as for cleaning and oiling (Beier, 1970).

So far, little has been written on springtails as food animals, but two mistakes keep popping up in the recent literature (e.g., Zimmermann, 1982; Stute, 1989) based on a citation by Geyer (1957; 122) of writings of W. Wallner.

The genus name *Aphonura* is wrong; the correct name is *Aphorura*.

Aphorura armata is described as a Collembola species that can often be found in flower pots, and the animals "jump around in a lively manner, especially after watering." However, *A. armata*, also known under the valid name *Onychiurus armatus*, is a species that has no furcula and can therefore not jump around. To defend against enemies the *Onychiurus* species secrete a fluid from their skin. They are therefore unsuitable as food animals.

When vivarium enthusiasts are asked what kinds of springtails they breed, the answer is almost always, "White ones." Most likely, this refers to *Folsomia candida* of the family Isotomidae and less often to *Sinella coeca* of the family Entomobryidae, which both belong to the suborder Arthropleona; that is, the springtails with a longer body and a clearly segmented abdomen.

White Springtail (*Folsomia candida*)
Blind Springtail (*Sinella coeca*)

Description: For a detailed description the animal would need to be placed under microscope as was done with *Folsomia nana* in Fig. 18. *F. nana* looks very similar to *F. candida*. Only an expert can differentiate between springtail species. We limit ourselves to note that *Folsomia candida* reaches a length of 1.5-3 mm, is white, and has no eyes. Looked at from above, the whole body is of the same width. The females lay minuscule, spherical, light brown eggs close together in locations where they do not come in direct contact with water. The new hatchlings are about 0.2 mm long. They can be found in large quantities in actively fermenting organic matter, for example, compost heaps.

Sinella coeca is also white and eyeless, up to 1.5 mm long, but the body is more oval. It loves warmth and humus soil, and can therefore often be found in greenhouses, flower pots, and manure. Both species can jump a couple of inches.

Development Times: No precise information is available, but we estimate that the generations follow each other every 2-3 months. Especially *F. candida* reproduces well.

Containers, Substrate, and Equipment: Springtails can be bred in rectangular plastic containers from 20 x 10 x 8 cm; that is food storage containers, large petri dishes, or small plastic or glass aquariums

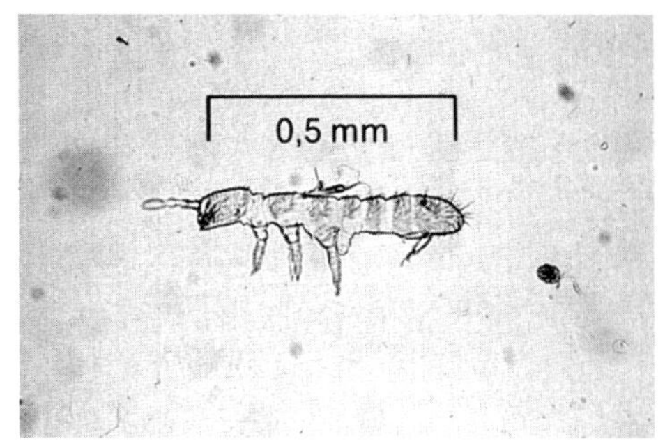

Fig. 18 The springtail *Folsomia nana*.

with a glass cover. Reusing food containers (ice cream, cheese, etc.) saves on expenses. The lid must be easily removable; the containers should not be airtight so that no air holes are required in the lid. Vertical, smooth sides are no obstacle to springtails provided the air is humid enough.

As a substrate, use fibrous peat, according to Biesôt (1988/89), 2/3 parts of peat mixed with old oak and beech leaves, chopped fern roots and a little potting soil, together with 1/3 part materials from insulating tiles made of cork, plaster, or according to Stute (1989) plaster; Mexifarn-tiles are placed on top. The peat is rinsed until it is saturated, squeezed firmly, and then put into the container, about 3 cm deep. When the peat has swelled up, the springtail breeding stock can be added.

A very thin slice of potato for food, and a lid on the 5-l ice-cream box (20 x 13 x 20 cm) complete the setup with which Horst Schlaile, Weissach im Tal, has been breeding springtails successfully for several years.

The cork tiles are cut into shapes with a carpet knife such that the one for the bottom layer fits exactly into the container, the two on top are cut out a little smaller so

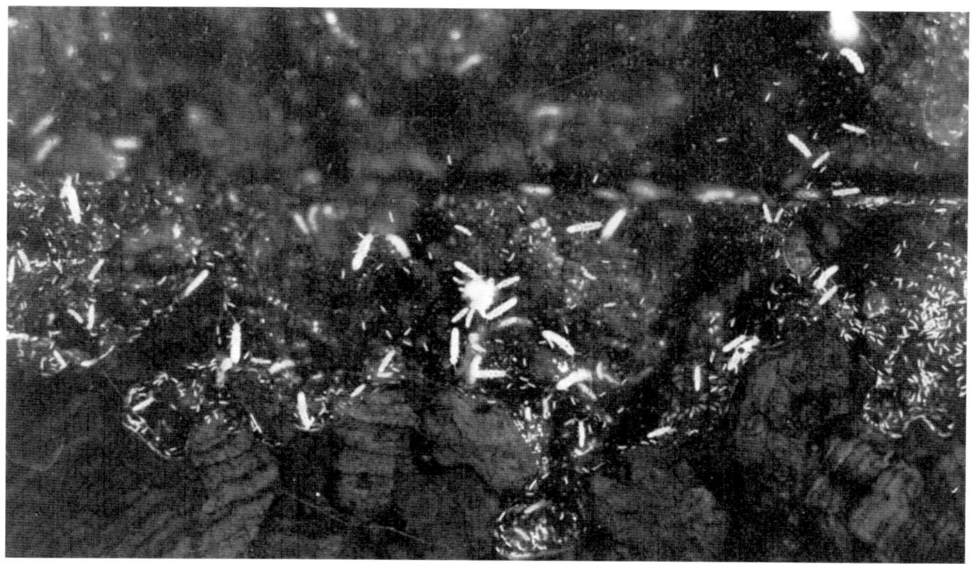

Fig. 19 Side view of a setup for *Folsomia candida* on cork tiles. In the middle some animals congregate around an oat; many young animals visible towards the right margin.

that they can be grasped easily. Spraying them with boiling water is the only other required preparation (Fig. 19).

To make substrate from plaster, mix alabaster plaster with water at a 1:1 ratio by volume (Wyninger, 1974). According to Bretz (personal comm.), the dry plaster is mixed with powdered charcoal (not chemically extracted charcoal) in a 1:3 ratio; according to Zimmerman (1982) it is mixed with activated charcoal. The charcoal binds to metabolic waste products, and the springtails are easier to see on the black substrate. The plaster is filled 2-3 cm into the breeding container. By drawing a knife through the hardening substance to create furrows, the surface area can be greatly increased.

If the inside of the petri dish is first covered with paraffin wax before the plaster substrate is added, the plaster can later be removed easily without breaking the dish by turning it upside down and tapping lightly on the sides and bottom. The liquid paraffin is spread around by gingerly turning the dish in all directions. The wax should completely cover the sides, the bottom, and the rim (Bretz, oral comm.).

Food: For the most commonly bred species suitable foods include thinly sliced potato, cucumber, zucchini, squash, carrot, or apple, as well as oats, brewer's yeast, baking yeast, soy flakes, wheat germ, ground up pellet food for crickets (Bretz, oral comm.), and rye flour (Schiller, 1989). Potatoes are the safest vegetable since the slices dry quickly and thus do not mold or rot like other vegetables if leftovers remain in the container after a few days. The pellet food as well as the yeast and soy flakes are preferred over potatoes, but they must be sprinkled more often in small amounts so that they are eaten before they have an opportunity to get moldy. Since it can happen that the mentioned dried foods already contain mites at the time of purchase, it is safest to freeze them for a few days before they are used.

If the springtails are collected outdoors (Rusek, 1971; Zimmermann, 1982)— for breeding or keeping—their first food should be the substrate in which they were found. Probably all these animals will also eat the green algae that grow on the bark of many trees. Small pieces of bark that are overgrown with algae can be added for the springtails to graze on.

Breeding Conditions:

Light: Since they dislike light, a dark spot is ideal for springtails.

Temperature: The breeding setups do very well at room temperature of about 20-22°C. Lower temperatures slow develop-ment. *Sinella coeca* prefers 25-28°C. Consider that there is more evaporation at higher temperatures.

Humidity: Most springtails prefer 100% humidity. The substrate should be moist, but not muddy or flooded.

Notes: The hardest parts of breeding springtails are to decide on a setup and breeding method, and the first three months. We will first describe Mr. Schlaile's method in detail, starting with an estab-lished breeding setup.

Five coolers form the basic setup. Every other day a different container is taken care of—after 1½ week it is the first one's turn again—in such a way that rinsing, misting, harvesting, and feeding of the springtails are combined. He pours a cup of water in the container and drains it over a fine-meshed tea strainer, careful that the

potatoes do not fall out. Since springtails swim on water, some animals will be washed out, too, and collect in the sieve. These can either be used as food, or returned to the container if it is not overpopulated. Then he adds a new layer of thin potato slices, closes the lid, and that's it! Sufficient leftover water remains in the container to last until the container is taken care of again in 1½ weeks.

With this method, leftover food is not removed; instead, the container fills up over time and the springtails live no longer in the peat he uses, but primarily between the layers of potato. It is absolutely necessary to rinse each container every 1½ weeks, otherwise the potatoes will get slimy. This method works using potatoes as the sole food item. The quiet period of 1½ weeks is necessary so that the animals can reproduce in peace. The setups are kept at a temperature of 21-22°C. The setup of the first container is described on page 62. The amount of food is increased as the springtail population grows, until the whole surface is covered.

All the other methods are designed provide the springtails with ample living space initially and to provide only as much food as can be consumed in 2-3 days. Leftovers are removed, or possibly left in for another 1-2 without adding any new food. Springtail breeding setups have the advantage that they can be left unattended for up to a month without feeding. They survive this easily but they will not breed during this time. It is important, that enough moisture is present. The containers should be watered thoroughly before they are left. Mr. Schlaile's setups survive his vacation time unattended. Upon return, thorough rinsing is necessary.

Each setup, regardless of the method used, requires special attention during the first few months (see "Pests"). The animals should be allowed to multiply from the breeding stock to a strong population before any are harvested for food.

After 4-6 months, the springtails must be moved into a fresh container.

Distinguishing between small-scale and large-scale breeding is not necessary since the only difference is the number, and possibly size, of containers. A guideline for the amount that can be harvested is that Mr. Schlaile harvests about 1 tablespoon of springtails from each container every 1½ weeks.

Pests: As in many types of breeding setups, mites can be bothersome guests, and also predators like the larvae of the sciarid flies and predatory mites. If the springtails are fed too much, the mites reproduce faster than the springtails and make effective breeding impossible. All methods for removing them, as for example, those recommended by Stute (1989), are a chore. We therefore recommend to restart any infested setup with breeding stock that is free of mites.

New breeding stock can be purchased, or some animals can be selected from a contaminated setup with the help of a strong magnifying glass and pampered back into viable breeding stock under strict control. Feed less on this second attempt!

Predatory mites (light-brown, actively roaming mites) cannot consume a large population, but a sparsely populate setup can be cleaned out. They should not be tolerated but dealt with as described above. Since they do not appear in large numbers like other mites, picking them off can bring results after a few weeks: Squash each mite (using fingernails and the sides of the container, or tweezers), and remove the vegetable or meat slices that attracted them. Sciarid flies get stuck on glue paper that can be hung from the lid. Their larvae live among the springtails and can be harvested along with them.

Fungal filaments (hyphae) cause a lot of damage to springtails (Mayer, 1957). The fungi grow over the food. This is another reason for feeding just enough so that the springtails will eat the fungi before they can spread.

A new setup is especially susceptible to the mentioned pests. Daily inspection of the containers, preferably with a magnifying glass, helps recognize the beginnings of any infestation and deal with it with little effort.

Feeding: If only a few springtails are needed, they can be harvested from the sides of the container. Springtails will also congregate in pieces of coarse fabric (e.g. sackcloth or nylon stocking) which are moistened and placed on top of the substrate. If cork tiles are used, they can be tapped to collect the animals.

Large numbers of springtails can be harvested by flooding their container, since they will float on the surface of the water. Horst Schlaile has incorporated this in his breeding methodology (see Notes). In setups with a solid substrate, the animals can be flushed by spraying it with a spray bottle, either into a bowl from which they are harvested with a fine-meshed net or directly into a sieve (for example tea strainer) that sits on a bowl. For all frogs of the family Dendrobatidae, springtails are an essential food. They are also important as a first food for salamanders, newts and other amphibians, and for most fish, especially those that live close to the surface, as well as dwarf chameleons and spiders.

Advantages and Disadvantages:

Advantages:

- Only microfood that is easy to breed for terrestrial animals
- Large-scale breeding requires a relatively modest amount of work
- High-quality food item
- Setups can be left unattended for 3-4 weeks

Disadvantages:

- Setups easily grow moldy or infested with mites
- Animals dry up quickly

Cockroaches

The archaic order of cockroaches (Blattariae) with about 3500 representative species has acquired a bad reputation worldwide as unwelcome houseguests. Worth mentioning in this context are the oriental cockroach (*Blatta orientalis*), the American cockroach (*Periplaneta Americana*), and the German cockroach (*Blatella germanica*). However, most cockroaches, which are common in the tropics, live away from human residences and lead an inconspicuous life, mostly at night. Noteworthy is their flat, wide body shape, which indicates a terrestrial lifestyle. The head and first thoracic segment are protected by a shield. Many species have lost their wings; sometimes there is only one gender. With mouthparts that are suitable for both biting and chewing, they can easily process solid foods.

All cockroach females lay their eggs not singly but in double rows, densely packed inside an egg capsule (ootheca). The four species described here are ovoviviparous; that is, the ootheca is not deposited but remains in the female's body until shortly before the larvae hatch. If the ootheca is visible, then it is just being formed, which can take several hours. The finished ootheca is maneuvered back into the body, into a special compartment of the uterus (a breeding pouch), with the help of appendages on the 8th and 9th abdominal segments. If the female expels the fresh cocoon, which can happen under stress, the embryos will not develop.

Nobody can recommend with an easy conscience that the cockroaches named above should be bred inside any house or apartment since they are extremely swift, have tiny young, can climb the smoothest walls, and escape through minute cracks. An entirely different story are *Blaptica dubia*, the Argentine cockroach, and *Blaberus craniifer*, the Death's Head cockroach, both in the family Blaberidae, which have been bred for several years by zoos and vivarium enthusiasts. These species move relatively slowly, especially *Blaptica dubia*, and they cannot climb vertical, smooth surfaces. They are therefore easy to manage and are under appropriate conditions extremely suitable for breeding, even indoors.

More care must be taken with the Surinam cockroach (*Pycnoscelus surinamensis*) of the family Pycnoscelidae, and the green banana cockroach (*Panchlora nivea*) of the family Panchloridae. Both are faster than the Blaberidae, and Surinam cockroaches can climb glass and smooth walls after their 5th larval stage. Green banana cockroaches can only do this as adults, but are able to fly several feet. However, green banana cockroaches require so much humidity that they might stay alive for a few days in an apartment, but will not be able to reproduce. This could only happen in a tropical terrarium, where the animals are unlikely to become a pest.

The potential for considerably bigger problems exists with the Surinam cockroach since it requires less humidity and lives in the ground, be it the soil of flower pots, terrariums, or, as the name suggests, greenhouses. However, each species has distinct advantages that make describing how to breed it worthwhile: Adult *P. surinamensis* are so small that they can also be fed to medium-sized lizards. The even more delicate *P. nivea* is a special treat for chameleons and larger tree-dwelling frogs.

Argentine Cockroach (*Blaptica dubia*)
Death's Head Cockroach (*Blaberus craniifer*)
Surinam Cockroach (*Pycnoscelus surinamensis*)
Green Banana Cockroach (*Panchlora nivea*)

Description: *Blaptica dubia* (Fig. 20): At a length of about 4 cm and almost 2 cm wide, these cockroaches are a large meal as adults. The males are winged with a flattened body, about 3-5 mm thick, the females wingless, stronger, and 5-7 mm thick. The shiny black-brown body has a light spot on each segment along the sides. More ore less discernible is also a line down the middle. The wing buds can be distinguished by their reddish brown coloring. The rims of the scutellum and of

the wings become light to middle brown as the insect gets older.

The egg cocoon is honey-colored. The newly hatched nymphs measure 5-6 mm, at first whitish-gray in color, then dull brown after their chitin exoskeleton has hardened. They keep this coloring until their last molt and resemble the woodlice quite a bit. When they reach about 2 cm, the genders are easily distinguished. The wing buds of the male are about twice as long as those of the female. The antennae are about half as long as the body.

Blaberus craniifer (Fig. 21): This cockroach has similar good properties as a food animal as the previous one, but it gets larger so that it is of interest to keepers of larger lizards. Both genders reach a size of 50-53 mm; the powerful wings extend beyond the tail by another few millimeters to that these animals reach an impressive total length of up to 60 mm. The wings also cover the sides of the abdomen (18 mm wide male; 21 mm wide female) so that the animals appear 27-30 mm wide from above. Both sexes are 10 mm tall. The dark brown base color of the body is interrupted by dark yellow spots that form a pattern. The transparent wings and the scutellum are light brown, with a dark spot on the scutellum and medium brown spots on the front half of the wings. The antennae measure about 30 mm.

With a little practice, the sexes can be told apart easily. Viewed from above the female has a larger neck shield. On the underside of the abdomen, the large segments are fused to form a triangular shape in the females. The last segment of the male's abdomen appears narrower, set off from the rest, and divided into two lobes (see Fig. 22). As mentioned, the body of the

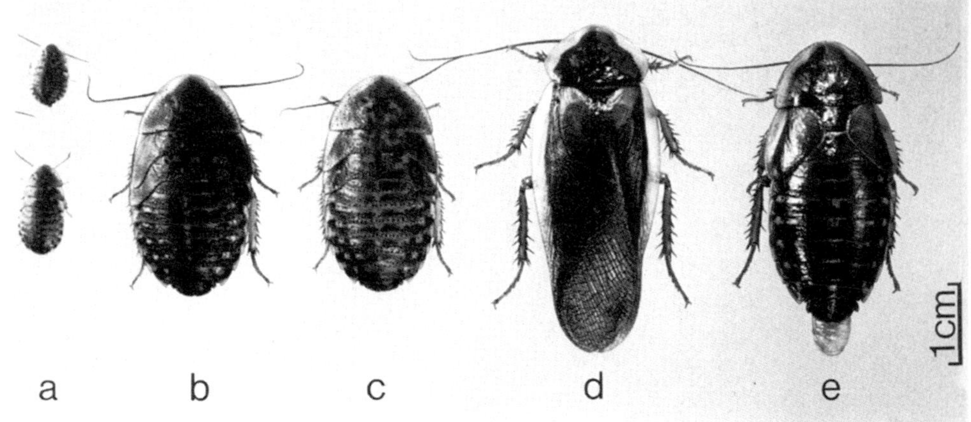

Fig. 20   Argentine cockroach (*Blaptica dubia*). a) Young nymphs, b) male nymph, c) female nymph, d) male, e) female

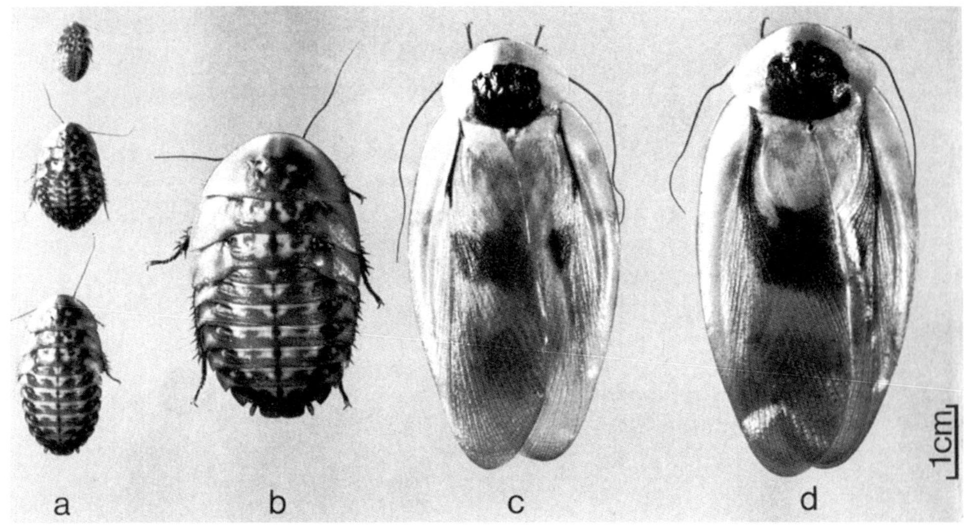

Fig. 21   Death's-head cockroach (*Blaberus craniifer*). a) Young nymphs, b) large female nymph, c) male, d) female

male is narrower than that of the female. This and the different shape of the underside of the tail-end of the abdomen can also be recognized in nymphs that are 4 cm long. With a little practice, even nymphs from 3 cm length can be sorted using this method.

From the dark-brown cocoon the nymphs

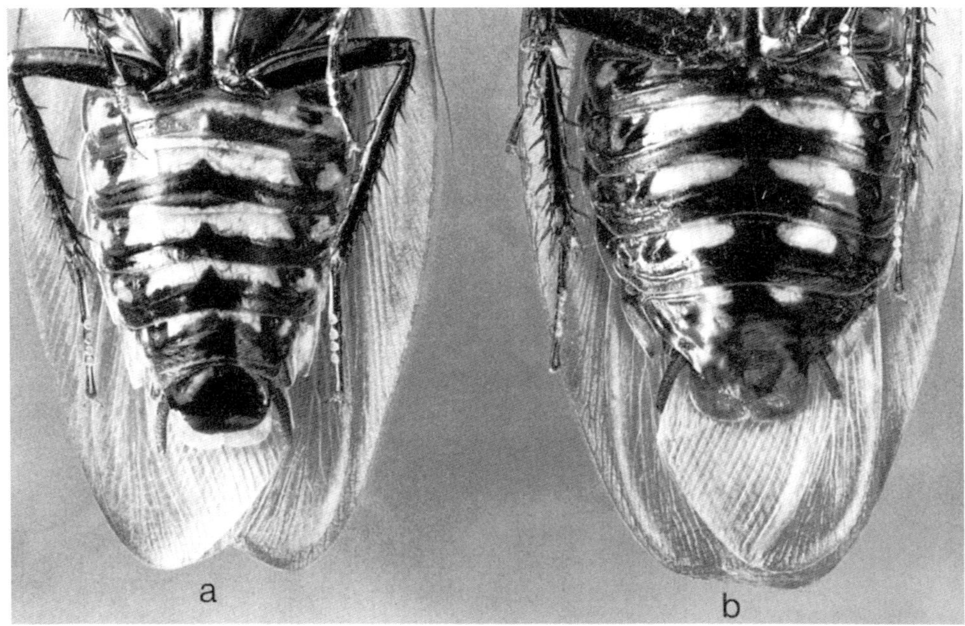

Fig. 22 Underside of *Blaberus craniifer*. a) Male, b) female.

hatch at a size of 6-7 mm. These small larvae managed to climb up glued seams and plastic surfaces if they are not completely smooth. They cannot climb glass. Unlike *Blaptica dubia*, the death's-head cockroach will secrete a strong-smelling fluid when touched. Many predators will avoid it because of this, but some prefer it.

Pycnoscelus surinamensis (Fig. 23): The Surinam cockroach reproduces exclusively through parthenogenesis: females only produce more females. Adult animals measure 20-28 mm in length, 8-9 mm in width, and 3-4 mm in height; the base color is brown. On the back, each segment has a lightly colored rear and side rim so that light, triangular markings become visible when the animal lifts its red to grey brown wings. The last two segments are black-brown, as are the scutellum and the head.

The antennae are 1 cm long. The wings almost cover the abdomen. The bristles on the legs are short and relatively soft. The freshly emerged nymphs measure about 4 mm. They glisten red-brown; only the last 5 abdominal segments are dull. Their original home is the islands of the Malayan Archipelago, where *P. surinamensis* probably branched off a bisexual form that has its own designated species today, *Pycnoscelus indicus* (Roth, 1967).

Today, *P. surinamensis* can be found worldwide; our breeding stock is from Florida. One common name that is sometimes used (greenhouse cockroach) indicates where this cockroach can be found most often when introduced into temperate climate locations; it travels unnoticed in the root balls of plants. Since

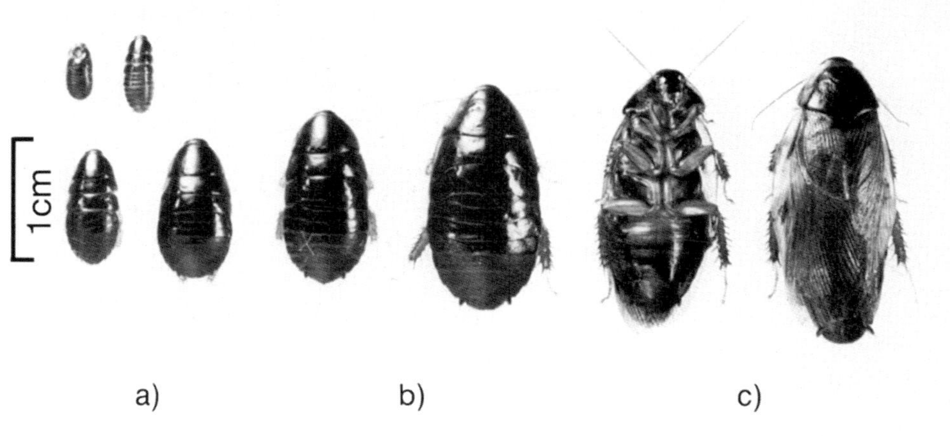

Fig. 23 Surinam cockroach (*Pycnoscelus surinamensis*). a) Young nymphs, b) large nymphs, c) female.

it lives in the upper layers of the ground, it was only discovered when research was done to find out, why, for example, rose bushes would not thrive: The cockroaches had damaged the subterranean parts of the trunk and the roots. In warm countries they can also be found in the open, for example, in potato fields (Hoffmann, 1927).

Panchlora nivea (Fig. 24): Even people who find all cockroaches despicable will look at *P. nivea* without disgust. The delicate, light-green animals do not fit the general idea of a cockroach. The body of the females measure 19-21 mm, is about 8 mm wide, and 2-3 mm tall; that of the male 15 mm long and 6-7 mm wide. The abdomen is rimmed by a narrow, whitish-yellow stripe. The rim continues on the front wings and the scutellum as a light marking that follows the outline of the body. The transparent wings and the scutellum extend a little beyond the body laterally, and about 4 mm in the rear. The antennae are 13 mm long and light brown. On the head, across the eyes, is a dark brown band. The underbelly and the fine bristles on the legs are whitish green. The egg cocoon is curved, thin-walled, and almost colorless. The nymphs measure about 3 mm after they emerge, are narrow at the head and wide at the tail, almost triangular, and light brown, later dark red-brown. They can only be distinguished from *P. surinamensis* by some greenish color on the underside.

Panchlora nivea originates in the Netherlands Antilles, Mexico, Central America, and South America. It is one of those tropical cockroaches that can only be found outdoors and do not survive in houses (Roth and Willis, 1958). Little is known about its biology.

70

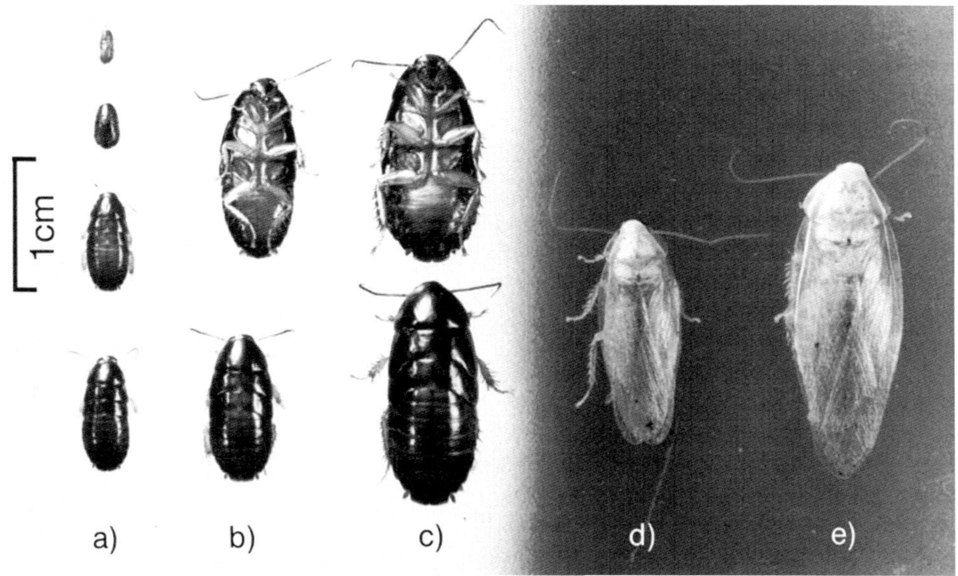

Fig. 24 Green banana cockroach *(Panchlora nivea)*. a) Small nymphs, b) male nymph, c) female nymph, d) male, e) female.

Development Times: *Blaptica dubia*: At a temperature of 23-25°C the nymphs require about 6 months to reach their last molt; at 28-32°C only 6½-9½ weeks. About 6 weeks later they are sexually mature.

Their life span is 1-1½ years. About 15-30 nymphs hatch from the ootheca. If a female is kept at a constant temperature of 23-25°C, she deposits a cocoon every 7-8 weeks. During the hatching, the female stands protectively over the egg capsule until all the young have crawled away in different directions; this can be considered a basic form of caring for the young.

Blaberus craniifer: This species is more fertile than the Argentine cockroach. One ootheca contains 34 eggs in average. At 25-27°C the female drops a cocoon every 3-4 weeks, and the nymphs reach adulthood and sexual maturity in 4-5 months. However, nymph mortality is rather high, only 55% reach sexual maturity (Willis et al., 1958). Life expectancy is one year.

Pycnoscelus surinamensis: At 22-25°C the larvae reach adulthood in 5½ months and reproduce for the first time 2 months later; at 30°C after 4-4½ months and 40 days. This cockroach packages and average of 26 eggs into the ootheca, from which about 20 nymphs hatch in the first reproductive cycle. One female reproduces 3-4 times. Adult Surinam cockroaches live about one year (Willis et al., 1958, personal observations).

Panchlora nivea: At 24°C the male nymphs require about 5 months to reach adulthood, females about 6½ months. At a constant temperature of 28-30°C this shortens to 2½-3 months (W. Schmidt, written communication). Six days after the molt that precedes sexual maturity, the females are ready to mate; two months later, the first young hatch. About two months later the females reproduce again, rarely a third time. These times were measured at 24°C. From one ootheca 28-60 larvae, 46 in average, hatch (Roth and Willis, 1958).

Container, Substrate, and Equipment: Any smooth-sided container with a tightly closing lid is suitable for housing purposes, such as a glass or plastic aquarium, a bucket, or a household tub. For ventilation, most of the lid should be made of screen, except for *P. nivea*, where smaller openings are better to keep the moisture in. Especially suitable is a container with a wire-mesh bottom through which excrements fall, which makes cleaning a lot easier. Examples of such a setup are a home-built box (Fig. 25) or a plastic tub whose bottom has been cut out, covered with screen (2-2.5 mm mesh), and reinforced with a larger-meshed wire-mesh. The tub is placed on blocks in a matching tray. About 800 cm^2 (e.g., 20 x 40 cm) suffice for 300-500 animals, 1600 cm^2 for 700-1200 animals. The container should be 15 cm high. This is not high enough for the Surinam and the green banana cockroach, where it should be at least 20 cm high. For these two species, a container with a wire-bottom cannot be used, as they require large amounts of substrate.

The "furnishings" for *Blaptica dubia* consist of several large egg cartons in layers, with one area of the enclosure left clear for feeding the moist food. For *Blaberus craniifer* a 2 cm layer of wood shavings or unfertilized peat moss that is kept slightly moist have shown to be good

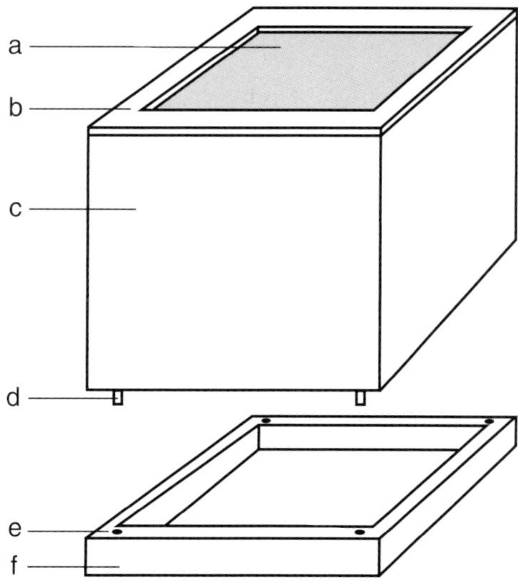

Fig. 25 Cockroach breeding box made of PVC. a) Wire mesh, b) lid, c) breeding container with wire-mesh bottom, d) feet, e) holes for feet, f) tray.

substrates; the egg cartons are placed on top. Surinam cockroaches like to dig into deeper, structured, and lightly most soil. Coarse, fibrous peat moss is the only or primary substrate, which can be mixed with compost, wood shavings, rotting wood or ground up bark. Unfertilized potting soil with clay or Bentonite clay is also suitable. This layer should be at least 5 cm high, better 10-20 cm. On top comes a piece of bark or an egg carton. For the green banana cockroach, a good substrate is plain peat moss or peat moss mixed with leaf litter, bark mulch, or partially composted leaves. This substrate must be kept very moist, almost wet, and filled in loosely to about 5 cm. On top come 2 layers of egg cartons, densely packed, pressed slightly into the soil.

It is important that all the containers can be

maintained from above since the cockroaches, which do not like light, will congregate underneath the egg cartons and, especially if the population is large, they can fly away through an opening in the side. Breeding will not be very successful at just room temperature. The following can be used to provide additional heat: Space heaters, tiled stove, lamp ballast, heat tape or heating pad, infrared heat emitter, or a climate-controlled cabinet. (Heat tape or heating pad should be placed inside a false bottom so that the cockroaches cannot damage any of the wiring.)

Food: Most cockroaches are omnivores. Since their stomach contents are passed on to the vivarium animals, they should be spoiled a little. Suitable dry foods are oats and puppy flakes, flake food for fish, wheat germ, cricket pellets, pellets for chickens, rabbits, cats, fish, or mice. Some pellets are very hard and the cockroaches have difficulties eating them. They can be coarsely ground. This dry food is simply sprinkled into the container or on top of the egg cartons for the two Blaberidae species, for the Death's Head cockroach only between the egg cartons. If the container has a wire-mesh bottom, the food is of course only sprinkled on the egg cartons. The Surinam cockroaches get both their dry as well as their moist food underneath the bark piece directly on the substrate. Since for these breeding setups mites are a most unpleasant pest, and much prepared animal food will develop mites, you should make a habit of removing all old food completely before new food is offered (Ulrich Ziegler, oral communication). The green banana cockroaches are fed a few pellets or a spoonful of oats in a couple of places directly on the substrate where the food will quickly become soft.

The always-present threat of mold dictates careful feeding. In general, all dry foods should be given sparingly; it should be completely eaten at the latest after a week. Wheat germ dries out especially fast. Drinking water is not required if the diet is rich in moisture. The water requirements are satisfied by offering moist food that is given fresh every 1-2 days. Remove leftovers first! This food is placed in a shallow dish on the bottom of the breeding container, on the bottom directly, or on the substrate. Dandelion greens, Endive, apple, orange, carrot, cooked rice, softened grain, quark, and prepared baby cereals are a selection of foods that can be fed all year for a varied diet.

Green banana cockroaches prefer fruit, especially oranges and bananas, and the adults require honey, which is dripped onto the egg carton or offered in a shallow dish. Once the setup is established, green banana cockroaches need only be fed once a week.

Breeding Conditions:

Light: cockroaches love darkness and are nocturnal. Therefore, a dark location is perfect for them. However, it is preferable if they get some light for a few hours a day so that they become inactive.

Temperature: The discussed species only are comfortable at temperatures around 25-30°C and reproduce well at those temperatures. The maximum temperature should be only a little above 30°C, since at extended exposure to temperatures around 35°C they will fall into a heat-induced stupor and die eventually (Beier, 1974). This explains why some breeders noticed that *Blaptica dubia* did not reproduce any more at 33-34°C. At temperatures below 15°C, the cockroaches will not reproduce either. At

5°C *P. surinamensis* will die (Zappe, 1918; Saupe, 1929).

Humidity: Air humidity should not fall below 80% for the green banana cockroach, not below 60% for the death's-head cockroach, and not below 50% for the Surinam cockroach. For Argentine cockroaches, 30-40% is sufficient.

Notes: Large-scale breeding is only different in the number and sizes of breeding containers. Cockroaches are, except for *Panchlora nivea*, very easy to breed. Because of their long lifespan and their slow development, breeding progresses continuously and without large fluctuations, unlike migratory locusts. This is why breeding cockroaches is also suitable for the vivarium enthusiast who only keeps a few animals, since with cockroaches, some food will always be available. Especially *Blaptica dubia*, which is the slowest moving of the four species, is almost ideal for breeding in an apartment and can almost completely replace mealworms. We know of no case where escaped cockroaches could take a hold or reproduce in an apartment that was kept at a commonly accepted level of cleanliness. They can get by without food for weeks, but will get weaker and weaker, and eventually any escapee will be found completely weakened or dead. If necessary, traps can be placed. However, it is possible that the cockroaches will reproduce in a large terrarium that offers favorable conditions, such as warmth, food, and places to hide. It may be necessary to control them on occasion.

The breeding stock for *Blaptica dubia* and *Blaberus craniifer* should not have too few animals: 25–30 females, 5-10 males, and 50-100 nymphs of various sizes are the minimum. For *Pycnoscelus surinamensis* 30-50 specimens are enough, for *Panchlora nivea*, 10-20 pairs.

A single container is enough for small-scale breeding for *B. dubia* and *B. craniifer* if the container has a wire-mesh bottom. A second container to transfer to is required for the green banana cockroaches, and it also makes cleaning easier, which should be done every 3-6 months depending on population density. The most convenient time for cleaning is when all the food has been eaten and the substrate is dry so that it can be sifted (exception: green banana cockroaches). The fastest way to do this is to have a second container prepared. For the Blaberidae, every layer of egg carton is turned over and tapped so that dirt and excrements fall off, and then placed into the second container. (It is not necessary to replace the egg cartons every time). Then the substrate is sifted to remove excrements and dust. For containers with wire-mesh bottoms the egg cartons are turned around and on the next day, after all the debris has had a chance to fall down, the tray is cleaned.

For major cleaning of the containers for the two large cockroach species, and for each cleaning of the green banana cockroach, a large sieve is employed. It is best to work in two stages, first with a sieve that has a mesh size of 3-4 mm, then one with a mesh-size of 1.5-2 mm. In this manner, the adults and large nymphs, which will scatter when exposed to light, can quickly be moved to their new container. Never leave the sieve unattended as the adult Surinam cockroaches and their larger nymphs can climb over the rim.

Since the wet substrate of *P. nivea* cannot

be sifted, a different method must be employed. After the first cleaning, all adult animals are moved into the new container. In subsequent weeks, the nymphs that have grown large enough are rehomed. After a few weeks of this, all the nymphs will have grown large enough to be moved. For a while, the old and new containers are maintained in parallel.

Pests and Diseases: Known pests are several types of mites that are introduced with wild plants or prepared animal feed. Usually they will not eat the cockroaches, only their food, however, when they occur in masses, they disturb the setup.

We have observed two kinds of mites, which can be distinguished by their behaviors. One species, *Caloglyphus berlesei*, is white, about 0.5 mm big, pretty slim, and found all over the container: These mites sit and roam on the food, between excrements and debris, on the sides inside and outside and on our hands. Usually they can be removed by initiating a major cleaning.

In addition, the Argentine and death's-head cockroaches can be rinsed under lukewarm water in a sieve with tall sides. Only when they are completely dry (set on paper towels) should they be moved back into their cleaned container. The lid, the outer sides, and the area around the container should also be cleaned. Surinam cockroaches do not tolerate showering. (Their fear of water can be exploited to find them in flower pots: flooding the pot will force them from the dirt.)

The other type of mite, *Caloglyphus michaeli*, is beige, about 0.5 mm big, round, and can be found on the food, especially moist food, and excrements. Its presence is usually first announced by an unpleasant sweet smell that raises from the container. The leftover food must be removed with a large spoon since the mites will congregate there, and their nymphs can be found between the segments of the cockroaches. The mites do this, when there is a shortage of food. If conditions improve, they will drop off (Eberhard Wurst, oral comm.). It is incredible, how fast this mite reproduces and then appears in such numbers, that even the food provided for the cockroaches is not enough. At this point, they will also attack molting cockroaches, which endangers the whole breeding setup.

This mite has been found to be uncontrol-lable. For years we tried to control them (some nymphs always remain on the cockroaches), until good fortune came to our aid: Lesser mealworm beetles (*Alphitobius diaperinus*) got into our setups and ate the mites—so we suspect—at least after a while they had disappeared. Now we have to make sure that the beetles do not get out of hand!

The workgroup "Nieuwe voedseldieren" around the Belgian Peter de Batist suggests in their care sheets that the strong smell of the wormwood (*Artemisia absinthium*) drives mites away. They recommend to regularly add a tablespoon of this herb to the container to prevent infestation.

Since no wild cockroaches are fed, only captive-bred ones, no diseases are trans-mitted. Repeatedly it has been said that the gregarines (a sporozoan parasite of the family Gregarinidae) are harmful to amphibians and reptiles. This is not true and should be put to rest.

The low mortality of *Blaptica dubia* during its development is satisfying; are rarely there dead animals to be removed. What looks like large numbers of dead bodies turns out to be the cast off exoskeletons. Cannibalism only occurs if the population density is too large. Greater mortality must be tolerated for *Panchlora nivea* and *Blaberus craniifer*, but the latter are also more productive than all the other species. In the least favorable case, only half the hatchlings will reach sexual maturity if they are not used as food animals first.

Feeding: When feeding them it must be remembered that cockroaches flee brightness and will not come out of their hiding places during the day. Cockroaches are therefore offered to diurnal vivarium animals with tweezers (Surinam cockroaches are so round-bodied that they can barely be grasped with tweezers), or a needle, or in a smooth-sided dish (cover the rim with Vaseline for large nymphs and adults of the Surinam cockroach). If a cockroach escapes, it can be found in dark, warm hiding places, and should be caught. For nocturnal vivarium animals, only enough cockroaches should be put into the terrarium as can be eaten right away since they will quickly lose nutritional value. Chameleons are best placed on a close-by branch; if the animal is not interested in the cockroaches, they should be removed right away. With a green banana cockroach, this will rarely happen, as it is an irresistible bite. For water turtles, you should also make sure that the cockroaches are eaten right away so that they cannot escape to the land portion of the setup.

Many lizards, stronger amphibians, most water turtles, many small mammals, birds, predatory insects, and other arthropods (scorpions, bird spiders), and large fish that live close to the surface will relish cockroaches.

Advantages and Disadvantages:

Advantages:

- *Blaptica dubia* and *Blaberus craniifer* are food animals that can be bred in large quantities with little time investment; even more so than mealworms/mealworm beetles
- If fed an appropriate diet, high-quality and easily digested food; green banana cockroaches mostly as a supplemental food item
- Breeding setups are odor-free and there are no bothersome noises
- Breeding is worthwhile even if only a few vivarium animals are fed

Disadvantages:

- Cockroaches require high temperatures for efficient breeding
- Escaped animals hide immediately
- Many people are disgusted by cockroaches
- Green banana cockroaches are a little tricky to breed and less productive

Orthopterans: Crickets, Migratory Locusts, and Stick Insects

These insects are already familiar to most of us in two ways: the chirping of crickets reminds us so pleasantly of vacation evenings in the South, and the seventh plague to fall on Egypt brings to mind migratory locusts. These events already identify two major groups of orthopterans, which are essential food items for insect-eating vivarium animals.

One order, the Saltatoria (hoppers) with two suborders, Ensifera (long-horned hoppers) and Caelifera (short-horned hoppers), includes about 20,000 species. These are medium-sized insects with a thick head and rear legs that are adapted for jumping. They either lead a predatory life, eat plants, or are omnivores.

From the group of long-horned hoppers the crickets from the families Gryllidae and Phalangopsidae are introduced, which are grouped together in the super-family of the Grylloidea (crickets). Of the short-horned hoppers, all described species, belong to the family Acrididae (grasshoppers and locusts) and belong the migratory locusts. The second order, Phasmida (stick insects), has an illustrative common name. Most of the about 2500 species have a long, stick-shaped body. Many have large wings that enable them to fly in a more or less clumsy way. These nocturnal animals feed on plant leaves. Where they occur in masses in the tropics, imagine hearing the dripping of raindrops—but they are falling eggs that the females either drop or sling away. The two stick insects discussed here belong the family of the Phasmatidae.

House Cricket
(*Acheta domesticus*)*
Field Cricket
(*Gryllus assimilis*)
Black Cricket
(*Gryllus bimaculatus*)
Tropical House Cricket
(*Gryllodes sigillatus*)
African Cave Crickets
(*Phaeophilacris bredoides*)

Description: All crickets have a compact body with a rounded abdomen and hind legs that are strongly developed for jumping. If wings are present, the front wings are short, shorter than the abdomen, and the rear wings are thin and long, folded underneath the front wings and extending past the end of the body. The front wings are called elytra. The antennae are one-and-a-half to twice as long as the body, for the African cave cricket even three (female) to five (male) times. Newly hatched and molted larvae are whitish in their first hours of life.

The female can be recognized by her ovipositor, which is already developed in the mid-sized nymphs; it is split down the middle in old animals. Females use it to deposit their eggs one by one into the dirt, a little deeper than the ovipositor is long (10-17 mm). For courtship, the males of all crickets, except African cave crickets, chirp incessantly. They stridulate or sing by lifting and rubbing the front wings against each other. While they do this, a sharp edge (the scraper) at the base of one wing rubs along a filelike ridge (the file) on the bottom side of the other front wing, resulting in a series of "chirps." If many males are together, they chirp day and night, especially in the evening and early night hours. The male of the African cave cricket walks around the female with jerking movements and tapping at her with his long antennae. His wings are raised up; if he beats them abruptly forward, they generate low-frequency sounds that the females receive with their cerci (hearing

------

(Footnote: The name *Acheta* comes from the Greek and means "singer" and is of male gender. That is why the ending of the species name must be *domesticus*, not *domestica*.)

organs). Dambach and Lichtenstein (1978) describe the courtship behaviors of *Phaeophilacris spectrum.*

House crickets and black crickets have been counted among the easy-to-raise food animals for decades. In 1977, the tropical house cricket and the field cricket were added to the list (J. Rotter, written comm.). The African cave cricket has been known since 1968, but its use spread slowly and is only slowly gaining approval. Mr. Rotter also told me that the field cricket originates from a savannah-like environment in Ecuador and the tropical house cricket from Western Africa and Mongolia.

Acheta domesticus (Fig. 26): Domestic crickets are light brown with mottles that become dense enough to form a dark stripe down the back of the larvae; they also have a dark brown band between the eyes and the antennae. Adults measure 18-23 mm, and the females are in average larger than the males. From the 2 mm long whitish eggs hatch light, grey-brown nymphs of the same size.

The abdomen feels solid. Dead adults dry out.

Domestic crickets are very active and jump surprisingly high and far. Hungry nymphs are especially adept at jumping, mid-sized ones easily jump 30 cm! The adults, especially the females, like to fly and do it well.

Gryllus assimilis (Fig. 27): Field cricket. The adult field crickets measure 23-27 mm and are 8-10 cm in diameter. They appear brown, but when taking a closer look the head is light brown with a dark "m" between the eyes (looked at from behind), the neck shield dark, elytra and legs medium dark, and the abdomen black. The jumping legs have strong bristles.

Newly hatched nymphs look like those of the black cricket, only a little smaller. Older nymphs are grey brown to brown, always with a dark centerline on the abdomen and the typical mark on the head. The abdomen feels solid. Dead adults dry out.

Field crickets are relatively lazy; they do not jump wide or far. Similar to the house crickets, the females like to fly and can get quite far. In eastern Germany, field crickets are often called banana crickets. The species name comes with a small question mark, as its determination is not complete.

Gryllus bimaculatus (Fig. 28): Adult black crickets are 30-35 mm long and 12-15 mm in diameter. In addition to the black base color, the females have black-brown and the males gold-brown coarse front wings that show two light spots at the buds (*bimaculatus* = two-spotted). These spots can also be seen on newly hatched animals but disappear after the first molt. The red-brown jumping legs of the males stand out against the other black extremities. Black crickets, just like field crickets, look strong.

The eggs are 3 mm long, and so are the ant-like nymphs. The smallest nymphs are black, and with growing size they get lighter, light brown, and at first glance look almost like the nymphs of the field cricket. The dark head and single-color abdomen distinguish them however with a closer look.

Sniffing above a container with adult crickets, brings an unpleasant odor to the nose—they smell as if they were sweating. Their abdomen is quite soft at all stages. Dead animals turn mushy, which is especially noticeable in adults.

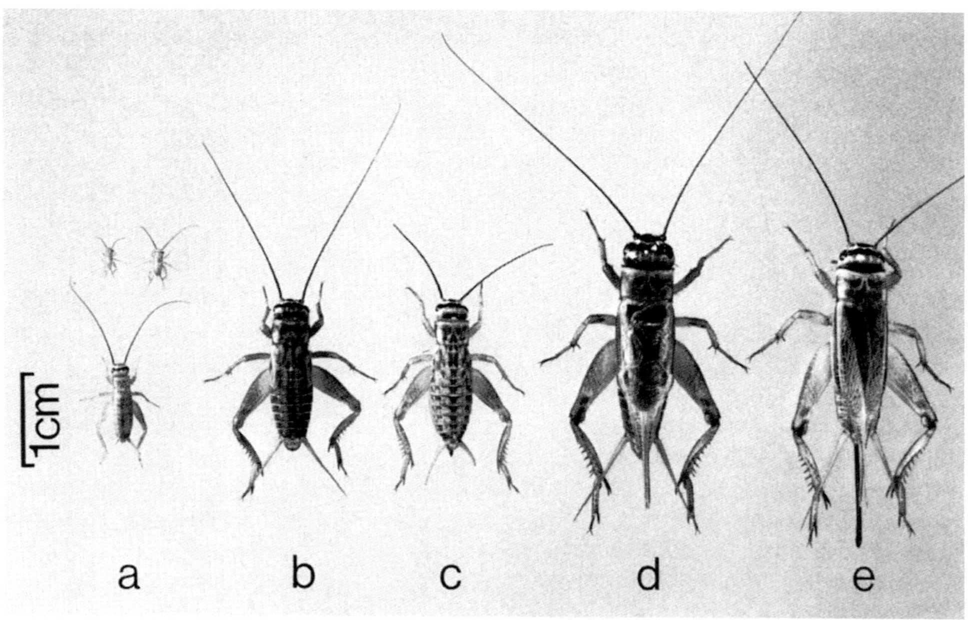

Fig. 26 House cricket (*Acheta domesticus*). a) Young nymphs, b) male nymph, c) female nymph, d) male, e) female.

This cricket jumps moderately, similar to the field cricket. However, the adults can fly very well provided they are warm enough. This is experienced particularly when trying to catch an escaping animal. Black crickets are out more often during the day than house crickets.

Gryllodes sigillatus (Fig. 29): The cricket is widely spread in the tropics and is mostly found near human habitation; thus its common name, "tropical house cricket." This delicate cricket remains at 17-22 mm length and 6 mm diameter smaller than the domestic cricket. When looking at the light brown, lightly mottled animals, a dark band over the first segment of the abdomen can be seen on female and young animals; in males, this is covered by the front elytra. Both wings of the female are reduced to small scales, in the males only the rear wings. A second, narrower dark band frames the rear of the scutellum, the third one, even fainter, connects the eyes. The legs are very lightly colored and transparent. From the 2 mm, yellowish eggs hatch nymphs of the same size; they are gray during the first days of life.

The abdomen feels soft. Dead animals dry out.

Phaeophilacris bredoides (Fig. 30): This African cave cricket was collected in 1968 by Dobroruka in the Chipongwe caves in Zambia, caves that are also inhabited by bats. He first described it as *Pholeogryllus geertsi* (Dobroruka, 1972). Kaltenbach recognized that it was not that species but a new, undescribed one, which he named *bredoides*. *Phaeophilacris* is the older

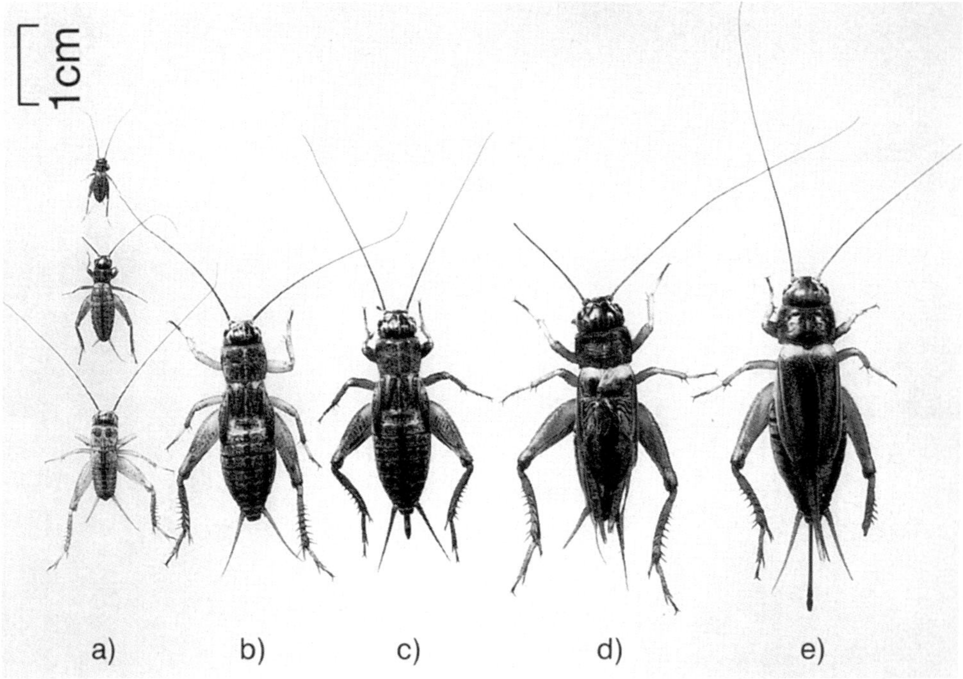

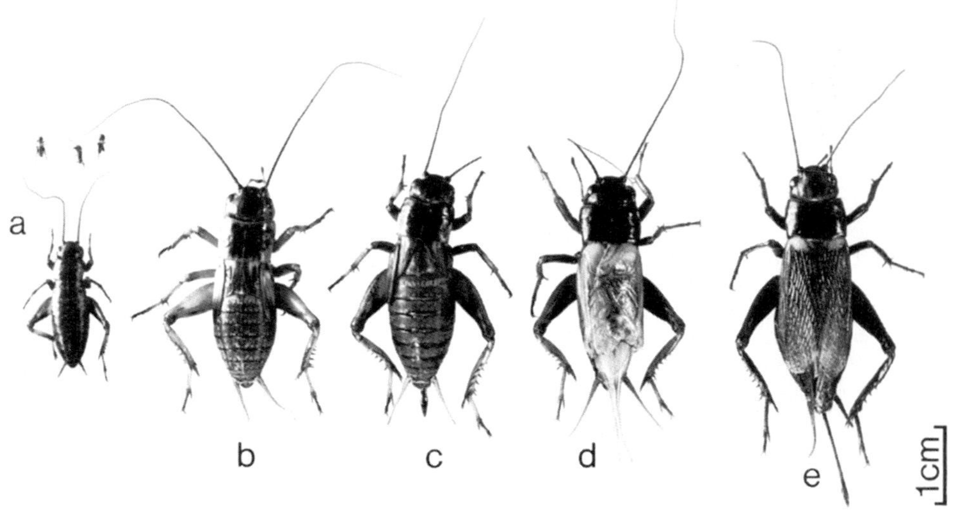

Fig. 27 Field cricket (*Gryllus assimilis*). a) to e) see Fig. 26.

Fig. 28 Black cricket (*Gryllus bimaculatus*) a) to e) see Fig. 26.

80

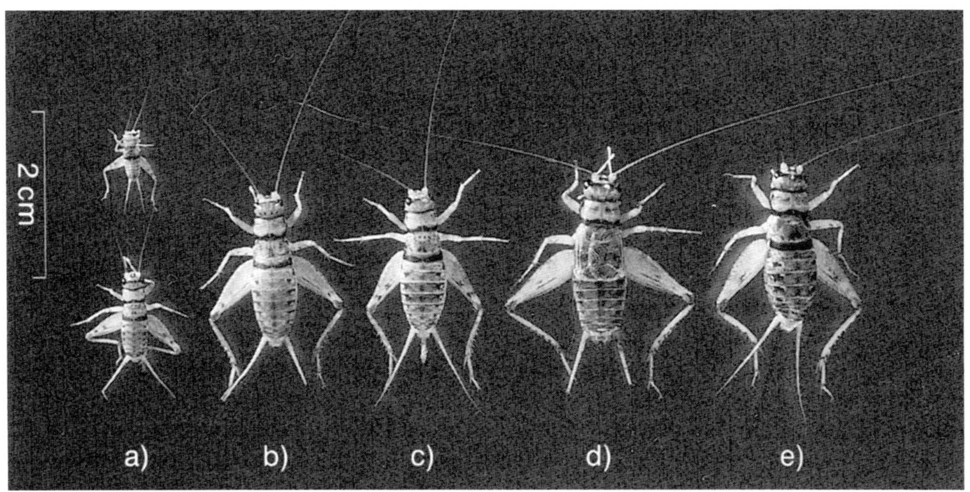

Fig. 29 Tropical house cricket (*Gryllodes sigillatus*). a) to e) see Fig. 26.

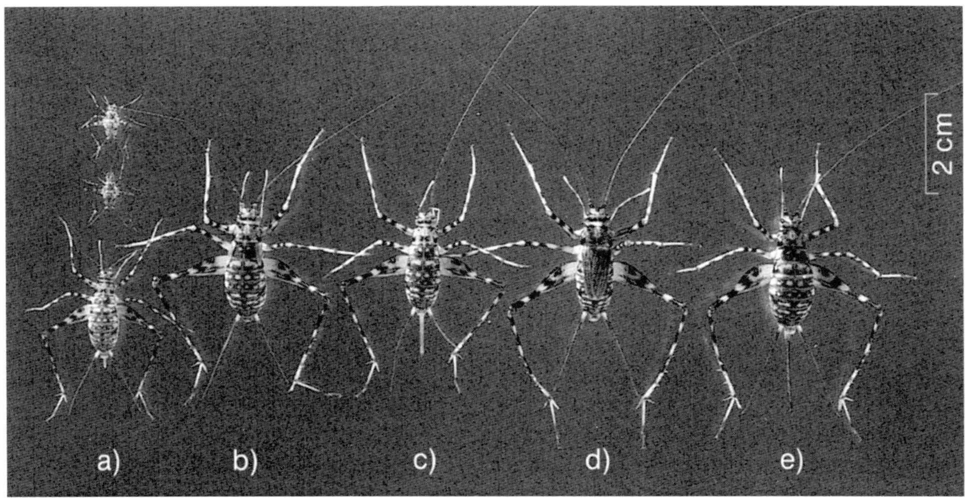

Fig. 30 African cave cricket *(Phaeophilacris bredoides)*. a) to e) see Fig. 26.

valid genus name.

The females are at 19-24 mm length, 7-9 mm diameter, and 8-10 mm height usually a little larger than the males at 18-23 mm length and 5-7 mm diameter.

The difference between the sexes is striking. The females' distended abdomen is widest where the jumping legs attach. There are not rudimentary wings. Instead, two small scales cover the abdomen. The front one is very small and easily over-looked; the rear one is dark brown and usually displays a small brown spot near the center and at the front rim. A thin light line runs along the center of the back. The body of the males is all the same width and is straight. The elytra are rounded and cover two thirds of the abdomen.

African cave crickets are light brown with darker markings and light/dark banded legs. The scutellum has two dark spots on the front rim and three on the rear rim, and on the sides, each has a washed out spot. Such washed out brown spots also appear on the head, from the eyes and the antennae down to the mouthparts. The underside is light. The extremely long rear legs (about 5 cm in adults), stick up and out, as far again as the body, and the distance between the knee joints is 2.5-3 cm in adults. The two pairs of front legs are also very long. The bristles on the legs are quite long but relatively soft. Eggs and newly hatched grey-brown larvae are round and 3 mm long.

The African cave crickets smell rather strong. Their abdomen feels soft.

The long rear legs with their strong thighs leave no doubt that these are strong jumpers.

In the following sections, the term "crickets" refers to all the mentioned species, unless a species is mentioned specifically.

Development Times: *Acheta domesticus:* The incubation period of the eggs at 20°C is about 21 days, at 25°C 14 days, and at 30-33°C 9-10 days. At 25°C the larvae reach adulthood in 5-6 weeks, at 30-33°C in 4 weeks. A female pro-duces 200-300 offspring in its 12-week life.

Gryllus assimilis: At 25°C the young crickets will hatch in 13 days, at 30-33°C in 9 days. The development to adulthood takes 6-7 weeks, resp. 5 weeks, at the above temperatures. The number of offspring per female is 250-350. The females live about 12 weeks.

Gryllus bimaculatus: At 25°C the larvae hatch in 12 days, at 30-33°C in 8 days. To fully develop the nymphs require 8 weeks at 25°C, 5-6 weeks at 30-33°C. In the course of her 6-week life, a female pro-duces 200-300 offspring.

Gryllodes sigillatus: At 22°C the nymphs hatch after 22-25 days, at 25°C in 16 days, at 28-31°C in 14 days. They reach adulthood in 8-9 weeks at a temperature of 22°C, in about 7 weeks at 25°C, in 5 weeks at 28-31°C. Every week a females produces 250-300 offspring, and that for its whole life, which is about 6 weeks, which makes for a total of 1500-1800 animals!

Phaeophilacris bredoides: At a room temperature of 20-22°C the development takes a long time: The nymphs hatch after about 8 weeks and reach adulthood in 9-10 months. At 26-27°C the succession of generations shortens to 5-6 months; embryo development takes about 3 weeks, the nymphs reach adulthood in 4-5 months; then they live for another 4-6 months. A female produces 150-200 offspring. Temperatures above 30°C inhibit development.

Containers, Substrate, and Equipment: Any container with smooth sides of at least 25 cm height is suitable; for tropical house crickets 30 cm height, for cave crickets 35 cm. Glass or plastic aquariums, storage boxes, buckets, as well as the cages shown in Figs. 31 and 37 are suitable.

For the African cave crickets, which like to jump, a box with a relatively small sliding door in the bottom half of the front panel is especially useful; or a cage for grasshoppers or stick insects with glass sliding doors can serve as a basic model. The optimal measurements for the animals and for running a well-producing breeding setup are 50 x 40 x 80 cm. Since these crickets like to sit head-down on vertical surfaces, their box should be covered with cardboard (rough surface to the inside). All containers require a tight-fitting lid; at least half of it should be wire-mesh with a mesh size of about 0.5 mm. For tall containers, a small, wire-mesh-covered ventilation opening on the side is recommended. The container for the black crickets must be especially well ventilated since the adults, particularly, do not tolerate high humidity.

The size of the container does not depend only on the number of animals kept and bred but also on the species and even the temperature (see "Special Hints").

House crickets and tropical house crickets tolerate the highest population density: about 500 adult animals can be kept in a box of 50 x 20 x 25 cm (Fig. 32). Only 250 field or black crickets would fit into the same container. If it was 10 cm higher, it could hold 75 African cave crickets. If animals of varying sizes are housed together, just about twice as many can be fit into the same container. For reasons that will be explained later, it makes sense to have at least two setups running. For a small breeding setup, a footprint of 20 x 15 cm per box suffices, only for the long-legged African cave crickets 30 x 20 cm are required.

Black crickets require constant high temperatures during the day and need a heater. If you do not depend on setups with uniform production rates the other species can be heated by ambient/external sources.

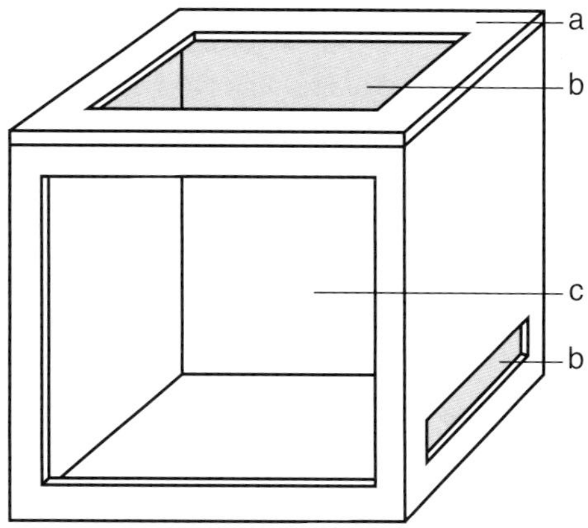

Fig. 31 Home-built cricket breeding container made of PVC or coated wood . a) Lid, b) wire mesh, c) frontal glass pane.

If the container is located in a dark corner, incandescent light bulbs can be used, otherwise, an infrared heat emitter or heat tape is recommended.

We recommend a shallow, 2 mm layer of sand or fine wood shavings for a substrate, or, according to Ehlert (1982), a layer of corrugated cardboard, so that excessive moisture can be absorbed. To be able to stock a container with the maximum number of field or black crickets, you can construct multiple "floors" made from egg cartons that are loosley stacked horizontally or vertically and loosely on top of each other for large animals, and interlaced for smaller ones. For house crickets, the egg cartons are broken into handy 10 x 10 cm pieces. Alternatively, cardboard tubes, for example, from toilet paper rolls, can be stacked. To enlarge the surface area, a second, folded tube can be inserted into each tube. For the smaller larvae, rolled up corrugated cardboard can be used. These tubes are mandatory for the active tropical house cricket. The animals feel pretty safe

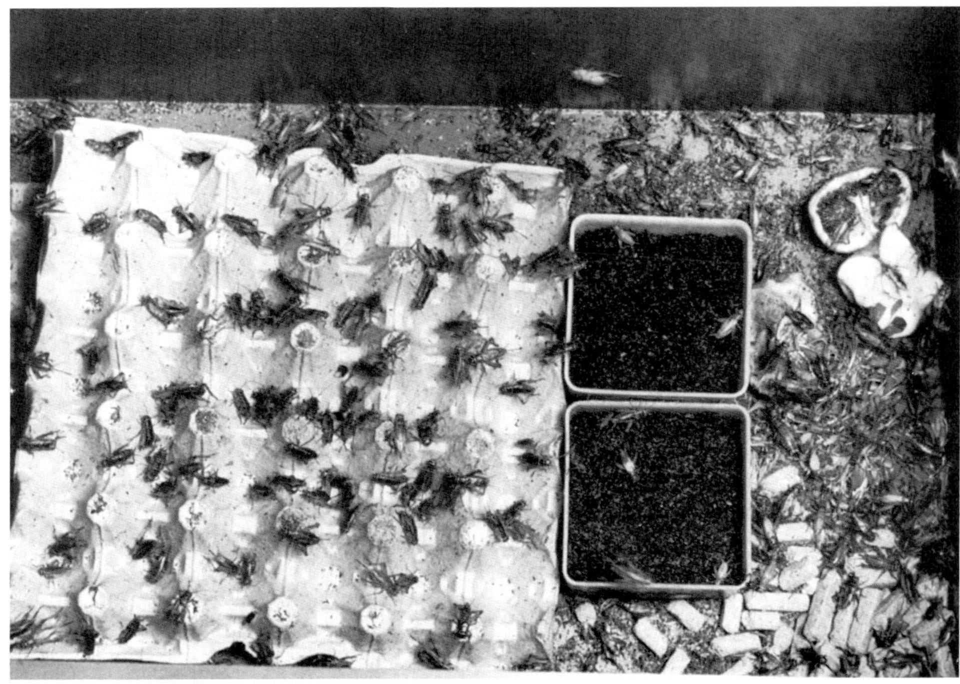

Fig. 32 View into a house cricket breeding setup.

inside the tubes and remain sitting in them when they are transported carefully, with calm movements. African cave crickets also like to sit in the paper tubes, especially if they are closed off at one end. In those the animals remain quietly seated—most of the time—when the tubes are moved. For the medium-sized larvae and adults single tubes of up to 12 cm diameter and 20 cm length are recommended to accommodate their size. Small cardboard boxes that have a 10 x 10 cm bottom area and 12-15 cm sides can be stacked up against the walls. When setting up the container, some room must be left for the egg-laying container and for feeding moist food. There should also be at least 10 cm between the substrate and the rim of the container for the crickets

that like to jump); otherwise, they will jump out when the lid is lifted off.
Cricket females lay their eggs into a moist substrate. For this purpose a can that measures at least 8 x 8 x 5 cm is filled with pure sand or lava sand (grain size 1-2 mm), peat, potting soil, or a mixture of equal parts peat moss and sand, up to 1 cm below the rim. The contents are moistened and must be kept moist, but not wet, at all times.
If the substrate is too dry, the females will dig and throw the substrate out, especially peat moss. Sponges like the ones used for flower arrangements, have also been used successfully. They are cut to fit into the can. This material stays evenly moist, but it can only be used two or three times.

The egg-laying can should be placed adjacent to the egg cartons so that the females can crawl in and later the nymphs can crawl out. A piece of cardboard can be added to serve as a small bridge. If the animals have moist food available at all times, then drinking water is optional, but they do like to drink. A bird waterer comes handy; it is placed on the bottom of the container and secured to the side with a suction cup holder, so that it cannot fall over but can be cleaned easily. The crickets would drown too easily in an open water dish, therefore a piece of foam material is fitted into the bowl; the foam material must be rinsed out frequently. Alternatively, a piece of wadded up toilet paper can be used, but it must be replaced frequently.

Food: Crickets feed on vegetable as well as animal matter. A separation into dry and wet foods has proven useful. Good dry foods are oats and dog flake foods, fish flakes, pellets of all kinds, such as for chickens, mice, chicks, guinea pigs, dogs, turtles, or crickets, as well as wheat germ. Pellets are placed on the bottom of the container, flakes are offered in shallow dishes (add a bridge for the smallest crickets) or in a designated dimple in the egg carton, so that food intake can be monitored. About every 2 weeks, the leftovers must be thrown out since they become too hard from the heat. The wheat germ can either be served in a separate dish or sprinkled in a corner of the container. Since it dries out very quickly and will not be eaten anymore, only as much wheat germ as the crickets will eat in one day should be offered. It is better to start with small portions, maybe one teaspoon of food for 200 smaller to medium-sized animals. Of course, not all kinds of food are offered at the same time, in turn. African cave crickets like oats especially. Soaked coarsely ground wheat and cooked rice are preferred moist foods.

Apples, carrots, and lettuces (no head lettuce) are the basic fresh foods. Following the seasons all sorts of fruit, like cherries, apricots, grapes, or oranges, and wild herbs like dandelion or plantain can be used. It is very important to make sure that all fruit and greens are free of insecticides and other harmful substances. For example, dandelion should not be collected next to a road. Fresh food can be offered daily or every 2-3 days. Greens dry out fast; orange slices keep best. Only feed a little more than can be eaten in a given time. Since especially the females of the black cricket like to lay their eggs into larger slices of apple, only offer thin slices. Of course, leftovers must be removed so that neither mold nor mites can take hold.

Breeding Conditions:

Light: The breeding containers can be placed in a dark or bright location. The light-avoiding cave crickets can be kept in the dark. At least for a few hours a day complete darkness is necessary so that the animals come out of their hiding places to eat.

Temperature: Thriving setups can be expected with 24°C temperatures. For the African cave cricket 29°C should not be exceeded, while the other species just start to get warm at that temperature. Above 33°C is too much heat for them. According to research by Merkel (1977), the larvae of *G. bimaculatus* grow best at a constant temperature of 27°C and on a diet that is made up of 30% protein. At 20-22°C the crickets will still reproduce, but the development times become rather long. At night, they all tolerate room temperature well as this represents their natural environment more than constantly high temperatures.

Humidity: Crickets like dry heat, so the containers should never be misted. The need for water is satisfied by the food they eat and the water they drink. Around 50-60% humidity is ideal; only cave crickets and all nymphs prefer 60-80%. To reach these values, they can be misted lightly every day.

Notes:

Small breeding setups: Even though house crickets cannot cause any real damage, they are counted among household pests and must be handled with appropriate care; this is also recommended for the tropical house crickets. If some basic guidelines are followed, they can be bred in apartments. The guidelines are as follows:

1. When the fresh food is changed, make sure no small crickets hide between the peel and the inside of the fruit; shake the fruit inside the container.

2. Work under a bright light and place the container on an uncluttered table or floor that preferably is of a contrasting color to the crickets; in this way, escapees are noticed right away. Usually, they are hard to catch and it might be better to kill them before they escape.

3. Before removing the lid, make sure no animals are hanging on to it. Female house crickets especially like to fly up and land on the underside of the lid. Never leave the open container unattended.

4. To harvest crickets, place a narrow-necked bottle on its side into the container. When enough animals have congregated inside, set the bottle upright and cover it with a piece of cardboard or your hand. Alternatively, place a small piece of egg carton in the container and pick it up later; shake the crickets off into an appropriate-sized glass—still inside the breeding container. The small container can be placed in the refrigerator for 10 minutes until the crickets are hardly able to move; then you can sort out the desired size.

These recommendations also apply to the other cricket species; however, there is little risk that they will become established in an apartment. Field and black crickets are much slower and easier to see because of their darker coloring.

Should some animals escape, the floor and walls can be searched in the dark with a flashlight. That is where the crickets will walk around most often. The heat from an infrared heat emitter or a heating pad that is strategically placed and a piece of apple for bait will attract the animals. Finally, any spider that has made a web close to the floor is an effective helper—she will enjoy the unexpected meal. If many animals escape, cockroach traps should be used.

As mentioned before, even for small-scale efforts two breeding containers are recommended, because the container with the eggs must be swapped out regularly. If a sand/peat mixture is used in the egg-laying container this is necessary at the latest after 2 weeks to prevent mites or at least keep them under control. If sand alone is used, the egg-laying container must only be swapped out every 4-6 weeks. By that time, the substrate is so contaminated with feces and egg shells that it starts to smell bad, and mold might form, which must not be allowed. Besides, after removal, it still takes another 2 weeks for the last eggs to hatch. The desired size of the crickets that are harvested for food determines how the 2 containers are stocked. However, it is important to single out the breeders in any case. Only large, strong specimens with complete antennae, wings, and jumping legs, as well as—for females—a complete ovipositor, should be selected as breeding stock. Since old females will often dig up eggs and eat them, breeding stock females should be replaced every 6-7 weeks.

All small nymphs, up to the 3rd molt, require a higher humidity than the larger animals, otherwise, too many will die. At first, the moist dirt of the egg-laying container suffices. After all the eggs have hatched and the egg-laying container is removed, the soil should be moistened daily. No standing water must remain since the smallest nymphs drown very easily. Be careful when misting: A spray bottle can emit a strong enough spray to jettison larvae out of the container.

Field crickets are robust and tolerant of variations in temperature and humidity. Many vivarium enthusiasts prefer to breed them instead of the black cricket, which is very temperature sensitive and generally susceptible to stress, which leads to a high death rate when the animals are shipped. Hoffmann (1973) has noticed that *G. bimaculatus* can be kept for several weeks at temperatures ranging from 5-34°C and tolerates daily variations of -1.5 to 20°C, but he kept the animals singly. The highest possible number of eggs per female for females kept alone— about 1000 at 34°C—(Hoffmann, 1974) is much higher than the realistic number in a breeding setup.

Black crickets reproduce by far the fastest. Breeders who need large numbers of freshly hatched nymphs or many small crickets will likely overlook the disadvantages of keeping this particular species; that the animals jump and move very fast. Our experiences lead to the conclusion that black crickets can also breedin houses and apartments under certain conditions, just like the house crickets. They are also strong predators. At the Frankfurt zoo they have been intentionally released in the insect breeding room and some large terrariums in order to control cockroaches, which they are doing successfully (R. Wicker, oral comm.). On the other hand, it can happen that larger specimens eat small or young lizards.

The chirping of male crickets is perceived differently by different people, from pleasant to extremely painful. African cave crickets are mute, field crickets have the quietest chirp, followed by tropical house crickets and house crickets. Black crickets are by far the noisiest. It is true for all species that that lonely (= escaped) males chirp much louder than animals that live in a group.

African cave crickets are not crickets that can be bred in large numbers with acceptable amounts of work. Since they are also beautiful insects that behave differently from "normal" crickets, they can be found in many insect exhibits. Those who do not have to feed a whole nest of starlings but keep just a few lizards, and who might also enjoy watching insects, will not want to miss out on the African cave crickets. Their exclusion from food animal breeding setups because of their long development times as reported by Arnold (1983) and

mediocre rate of reproduction is unde-
served. The notes for large setups are also
valid for the other four cricket species.
Large-scale setups: For a large cricket
breeding setup, it is preferable to use many
medium-sized containers. In this way, the
different stages of development can be
kept separate. A series of five containers
could be set up as follows: one container
with adult breeders and a 10 x 10 cm^2 egg-
laying box for every 150-200 females
(exchanged weekly); one container with
egg containers and hatching young; two
containers with larger nymphs; one
container with adults for feeding purposes.
Usually a separate room will be available
for the crickets and it can be heated to
about 30°C.

For a huge breeding setup, a heated room
is mandatory. In principle, such a breeding
setup is built up as follows: The egg-laying
containers are removed from the container
with the breeders shortly before the first
eggs hatch. Depending on the number of
hatching animals, the can is moved daily to
every four days to a new setup. Up to 4000
nymphs can be kept in an area of 40 x 30
cm. After a little more than half their
development time, the half-grown nymphs
are strained through two sieves, for the two
smaller species of 3 and 2 mm mesh size,
and of 4 mm and 3 mm mesh size for the
larger species. The three separated sizes
are each placed in their own setups. This is
necessary for several reasons: Even
nymphs that hatched on the same day, can
grow at different rates. The larger nymphs
molt in shorter intervals than the smaller
ones and are voracious. If many animals
molt at the same time, they cannot eat each
other and the losses are limited. Large
larvae require more space than small ones.

For handling of the animals, the same
guidelines apply as for small-scale efforts.
However, in a dedicated breeding room not
as much care is required if animals escape.
Because of the higher temperature they will
prefer to stay in the room so that they can
be caught again, or a couple of geckos can
be let lose every so often to clean up the
escapees.

Storage: For vacation times only the
tropical house crickets cannot be stored in
the refrigerator; even at 8°C several
animals died over the course of only 8
days, at 4°C, all of them died. Of the other
species, all stages from the size of a
housefly and larger tolerate 5 weeks at 5°C
without problems. The crickets are packed
into containers filled with slightly moistened moss or paper towels (air holes in the
lid!). Animals should not be packed too
tightly. Egg-laying containers with ready-
to-hatch eggs can easily stay in the cold for
up to 3 weeks. Once they are warmed up,
the first eggs will hatch after 8 days at the
earliest.

To store large numbers of crickets, over
1000, they must be distributed over two
containers if at 30°C one would be enough,
and they should be stored at 20°C. Crickets
perspire at low temperatures! In any case,
care must be taken to remove excessive
moisture by using sawdust, bran, or paper.
As little as 12 hours in a moist environment
are a death sentence for most crickets, even
if they are kept warm thereafter. Crickets
can easily be stored at 25°C for a longer
period of time.

Pests and Diseases: Mites are often
introduced with peat moss or food. They
are not dangerous for the crickets but can
be bothersome if they multiply much. To
prevent this, the breeding containers should

be completely redone two to three times a year. If mites, which like to congregate around leftover foods, are noticed, repeated general cleanings are often sufficient to control them.

Feeding: Only feed vivarium animals as many crickets as they can eat in a short time. In a sparsely furnished and tightly closing vivarium, the crickets can be dropped in directly. For fish, they are shaken up with water so that they sink and cannot jump onto floating plants. Otherwise, they are fed by hand, from a needle or tweezers, or from a smooth-sided bowl whose height and size must be appropriate to the cricket species. To feed house crickets and tropical house crickets from bowls their jumping legs must be clipped at the knee joint, otherwise they will escape. This is an unpleasant job but still better than an infested apartment or house. All crickets are delicacies for all insect-eating animals, including fish. Since they eat both plant and animal matter, they are a high-quality food. They are superior to wax worms for raising reptiles.

They are also imperative for insect-eating birds. They are also valuable food items for prosimians because of their high protein content.

Advantages and Disadvantages:

Advantages:
- High-quality food animals of medium size, together with tiny young offer a large variety of sizes
- Can be bred in large numbers all year
- Almost free of odor if kept clean

Disadvantages:
- The chirping of the males can disturb sensitive people. *G. bimaculatus* chirps so loud that breeding it in lived-in rooms can become torture (this can be alleviated by keeping the adult breeding stock in locked cabinets or other soundproof containers.)
- Requires relatively more time and daily care; or at least every other day
- *Acheta domesticus* is a household pest and the tropical house cricket has the potential to become one.

African Migratory Locust (*Locusta migratoria*)
Desert Locust (*Schistocerca gregaria*)
South American Locust | (*Schistocerca paranensis*)
Moroccan Locust (*Dociostaurus maroccanus*)

Description: The size and color of the migratory locusts depend on the environment temperature and the food they eat so that they are difficult to describe. A varied diet as well as high heat can change a dark brown into a light brown, or a washed out yellow into a brilliant yellow, and they also allow the larvae to grow larger. The hatching nymphs are whitish and soft. They keep their color, which they acquire after the chitin exoskeleton hardens, until their last molt.

The males of all migratory locusts usually remain 1-2 cm smaller than the females, and they change color as they age. The antennae are short in all species.

To deposit their eggs, females burrow a place for their abdomens 8-12 cm in the ground and create a small cavity by pushing out their legs and wings. The eggs are laid in double rows, horizontally or

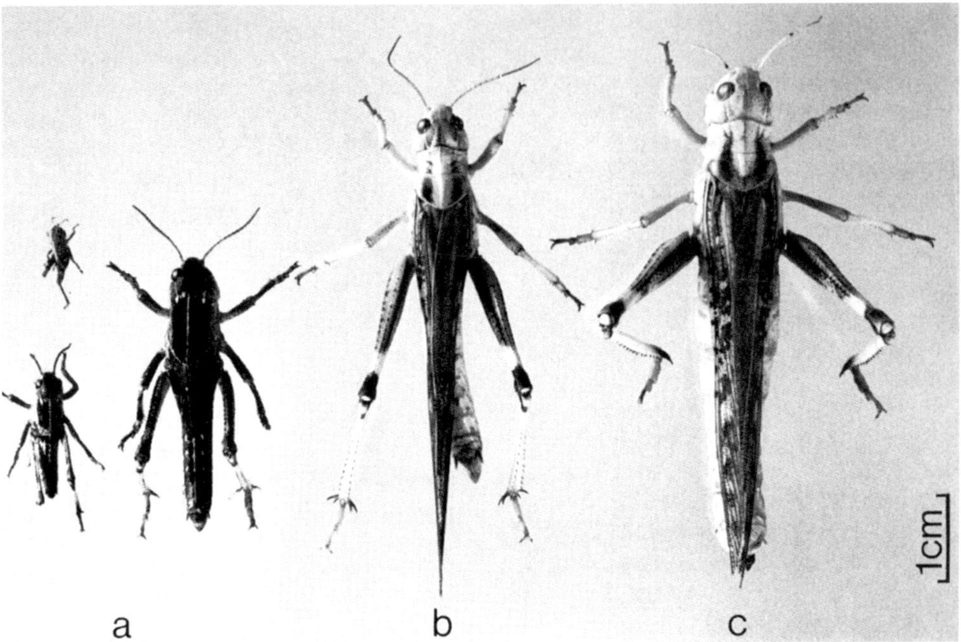

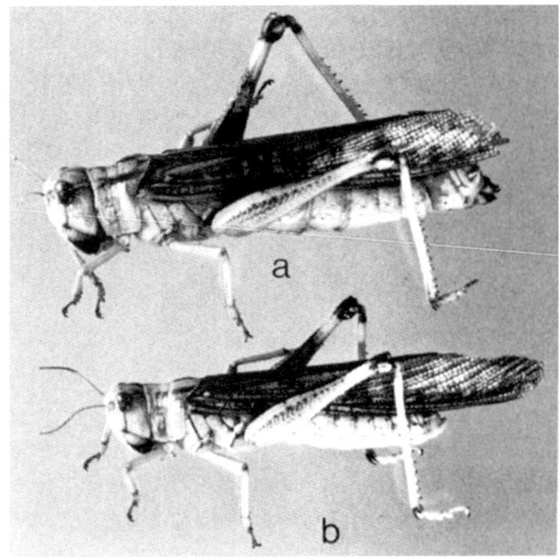

Fig. 33 African migratory locust (*Locusta migratoria*). a) Larvae, b) males, c) females.

vertically, inside a foamy secretion that is produced by glands next to their sexual organs. It takes 1-3 hours to create a foam nest that contains 30-80 eggs in this manner. The foam hardens and protects the eggs from drying out. During her 35-45 day adult life a female can produce 6-16 such nests.

Locusta migratoria (Figs. 33 & 34): This most commonly bred locust reaches a length of 4-6 cm. It is light gray to light brown with dark gray and brown spots; the wings are mottled light gray. The head and upper chest of the males turn yellow with age. When the larvae hatch from the 6 mm long large, elongated, light brown eggs, they measure 6-7 mm. Their blackish back is strongly set off from the medium to dark brown body. The African migratory locust

Fig. 34 Lateral view of African migratory locust. a) Female b) male.

90

can be found in Africa, Asia, and in areas of southern Europe.

Schistocerca gregaria: The adults of this beautiful locust reach 6-8 cm. Their coloring is dirt yellow, and their wings are dark brown and mottled. The larvae, which measure about 8 mm at the time of hatching and are as large as the eggs, are brilliant yellow with pitch-black spots. This species can be found in Northern Africa and occasionally in South America. Noteworthy is their calm demeanor while their container is being taken care of.

Schistocerca paranensis: This locust, which can be found in Central and South America, resembles *S. gregaria* in its coloring but stays noticeably smaller. Adults reach a size of 5-6 cm. When they hatch, the larvae measure 5-6 mm, and they are light brown or yellow with dark brown and black markings.

Dociostaurus maroccanus: An interesting and easy to breed species is the Moroccan locust. At 4-5 cm length, it is counted among the smaller species. Its base color ranges from light to red brown. A white stripe runs down the back from the chest to the tips of the wings. The eggs measure 5 mm and the 7-mm-long larvae have a light and dark brown striped pattern.

Development Times: *Locusta migratoria*: African migratory locusts are considered a classic among hopper food animals because they are easy to breed and have the shortest development time. A day temperature of 30-35°C and cooled at night to about 20°C, the larvae hatch in 12-16 days and are fully grown after 25-30 days. The adults reach sexual maturity 6-8 days later and mate. The females start laying eggs 4-6 days later. One clutch contains 30-40 eggs. After 7-8½ weeks a new generation has matured. If fed a varied diet the life expectancy of the adult animals is around 8 weeks. A female can deposit 12 clutches in this time period; that is, produce 360-480 offspring.

The development time of the animals shortens considerably if they are kept at a constant temperature of 30-35°C. To accomplish this, the lights must stay on around the clock so that their activity is uninterrupted. The larvae will already hatch after only 10 days, and they are fully grown after 20 days. Four days after the last molt the animals mate, and they lay their first eggs 3 days later. After 5 weeks, the new generation has already taken over.

Schistocerca gregaria: The desert locust requires a strong nighttime temperature drop of about 15°C. The daytime temperature should be around 35-40°C. Under these conditions the complete development takes about 9-10 weeks. The animals hatch after 18 days, take 30-40 days until they molt for the last time, and reach sexual maturity 10-14 days later. Egg laying starts 6-8 days thereafter. The foam nest contains 60-80 eggs; a female produces 6-12 clutches.

Schistocerca paranensis: This locust does not like too high a temperature; 28-30°C is ideal. If this temperature is maintained day and night, the South American locust has development times and reproductive rates that are comparable to those of the desert locust.

Dociostaurus maroccanus: The Moroccan migratory locust, like the desert locust, requires a change in temperature from about 35°C during the day to about 20°C at night. If kept at a constant high temperature the animals will die within a short time. A female can deposit up to 10 clutches containing 50-60 eggs each into the ground. The development times are the same as for *S. gregaria*, but the animals reach sexual maturity after only 6-10 days.

Containers, Substrate, and Equipment: Breeding cages can be custom ordered or homemade. Figures 35-37 show some models that have proven their usefulness. The large cages (e.g., 70 x 55 x 55 cm) are equipped with a stainless steel wire rack that can be inserted as a false bottom, and a drawer. Feces fall through the wire-mesh into the drawer and can be removed easily. If desired, the cage can be equipped with one or two sockets for incandescent lights or infrared heat emitters, and slats can be hung from the inside of the top to create more surface area for the larvae to molt. These types of cages are primarily recommended for large-scale breeding, where it is especially important to use an efficient setup that minimizes the time spent on maintenance.

Of course, such a cage can also be acquired or made for smaller-scale breeding. The following cage is well suited for a small setup and can easily be taken apart. The cage measures 40 x 30 x 30 cm and is constructed from 13 mm plywood or particle board. You need two side panels of 300 x 300 mm each, a floor of 375 x 295 mm, a back panel of 375 x 300 mm, and a lid of 375 x 100 mm, two u-shaped aluminum guide rails of 400 mm length each, and two that are 120 mm long, a glass panel measuring 400 x 174 mm, a glass panel measuring 396 x 116 mm, a piece of screen (1 mm mesh) measuring 400 x 210 mm, a piece of screen measuring 660 x 287 mm, an incandescent light bulb with a metal or ceramic socket,

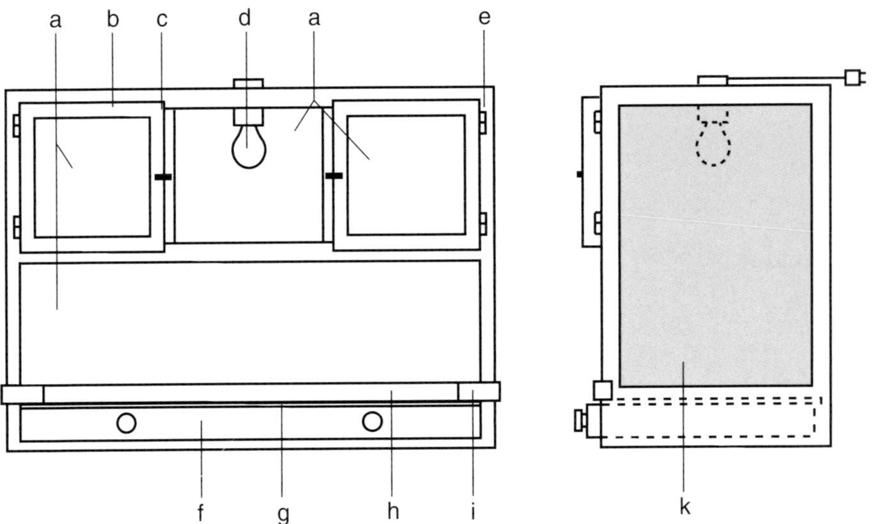

Fig. 35 Large wooden breeding cage for migratory locusts; front and side view. a) Glass panels, b) door, c) latch, d) socket with incandescent light bulb and connecting wire, e) hinge, f) drawer, g) removable wire shelf, h) sliding panel, i) angles, k) screen.

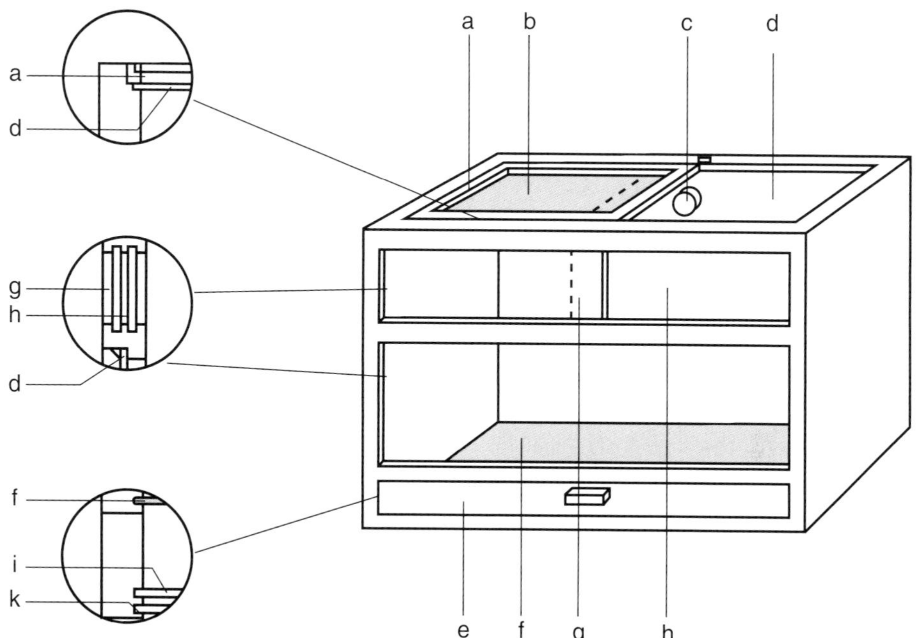

Fig. 36 Wooden breeding cage for migratory locusts. a) Movable wood frame, b) screen, c) socket with light bulb and cable, d) glass panel, e) drawer, f) wire-mesh floor, g) and h) movable glass panels, i) rails for drawers, k) cage floor.

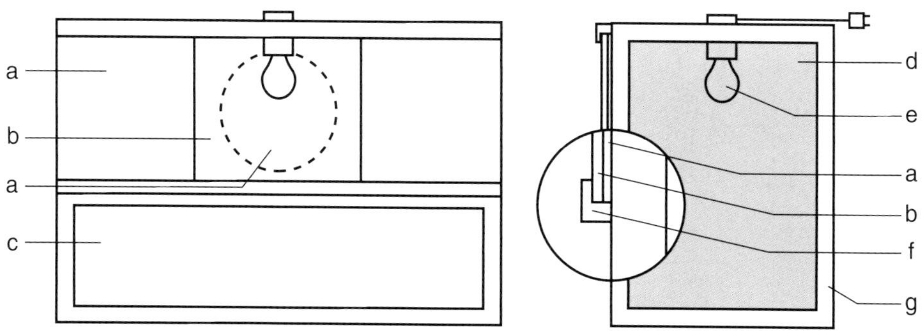

Fig. 37 Wooden breeding cage for migratory locusts; also suitable for crickets. Front and side view. a) Plexiglas panel, fixed, with round hole cut out, b) Plexiglas sliding panel, c) glass panel, d) screen, e) socket with light bulb and connecting wires, f) lower guide-rail, g) wooden frame.

wires, and plugs.

The cage is glued and nailed together. The bottom has to protrude as much as the aluminum guide rail for the front glass panel is wide. The 2 short guide rails are glued vertically to the front edges of the side panels, then you can insert the glass panel that must be flush with the bottom. For cleaning, this panel is pulled up and the feces can be swept out. The upper glass panel serves as a maintenance window which is opened only as much as is necessary for feeding and harvesting insects. The upper molding for this glass panel is glued to the edge of the lid, the other one to the top edge of the lower glass panel. To give the locusts enough space for molting and climbing, the inside of the rear and one side panel are covered with screen. The screen for ventilation is nailed to the edges of the side and back panel. The socket for the incandescent light bulb, which serves as a source of heat and light is now installed. This finished cage offers room for up to 300 locusts.

Freezer containers of 10 x 10 x 8 cm or similar containers are suitable as egg-laying containers. Only the desert locust *S. gregaria* drills its ovipositor up to 12 cm into the dirt and therefore needs appropriately tall containers. To allow excess water to drain, small holes should be drilled in the bottom.

The egg laying substrate deserves much attention, because the healthy development of the embryos depends on it. We have used a mixture of 40% well-washed sand, 30% leaf litter (leaf humus) and 30% unfertilized peat moss, all finely sieved, for years with good results. To loosen up the substrate, Styrofoam pellets can be mixed in. Eichner (oral comm.) uses bird sand with good results. Sand has the property that it retains moisture evenly, does not immediately respond to changes in temperature, and remains loose. Mixtures of forest dirt with sand, or sawdust with peat moss, are also suitable. Each breeder swears by his or her own recipe. Even more important than its composition is that the substrate is sterile and free of pests. To this end, it is moistened thoroughly, spread on a baking sheet, and heated to 130°C for about 15 minutes.

Food: If the locusts are to be kept alive as long as possible, they must be offered a varied and rich diet. As dried foods wheat bran, oats, dog flakes, wheat germ or ground up rodent pellets can be used. Pellets are especially recommended because of their high mineral content. In addition, old, not moldy bread or breadcrumbs can be offered.

The best fresh food is without doubt sprouted wheat (wheat germ), which is eaten by all species. The leaves of oak, beech, linden, maple, or plane trees, and all fruit trees, blackberries and raspberries can be offered, as well as vegetables and lettuces, especially endive, apple, pears, grated carrots, lucerne, dandelion, corn leaves, and many more. Lettuce is often covered with insecticide and is therefore not recommended. As for all insects, the food must be free of insecticides! Wash it well. Decorative bushes like lilac, laburnum, laurel, and elder have poisonous substances in their leaves and bark and are unsuitable for the locusts. All locusts like grass, for example the clump grass *Dactylus glomerata*, but there is a risk that certain nematodes might be introduced with it (see "Poisonings, Diseases, and Pests).

It is worth your while to grow your own wheat germ, not only for large-scale breeding but also for smaller setups. You only need a wooden frame covered with wire-mesh, which can easily be built (Fig. 38). To make the frame strong enough, use 60 mm x 20 mm wood. The desired pieces are sawed off, the longer pieces are screwed to the shorter ones, and a plastic or wire mesh with a mesh size of 5-10 mm is attached to the frame. At the corners, small wooden blocks are attached to the bottom to allow the air to circulate underneath. Different types of frames can be used, as long as the air can circulate easily.

The wheat can be bought from farm supply or health food stores and should be untreated, light-yellow, seed-quality wheat. The seeds must be scattered in a single layer on the wire mesh—for a frame of 50 cm x 30 cm about 250 g of wheat are required. The wheat is first soaked in cold water for 12-24 hours, then evenly distributed on the frame, which has been covered with two layers of newspaper. After 2 days the wheat begins to germinate, on the 4th day the roots have attached to the paper and the sprouts are 1 cm tall. They now grow up to 2 cm per day and can be used as food 8 days after the culture has been started (Fig. 39). They should not be allowed to grow taller than 20 cm since they will start to bend. For the duration, the sprouts are kept lightly moist and one day before they are used as food, watering is halted. Wheat germ that is put into the cages wet rots and gets moldy very quickly at high temperatures. In summer as well as in winter wheat germ can be cultivated in a well-aired room. If not enough fresh air is available, the sprouts will develop mold. A

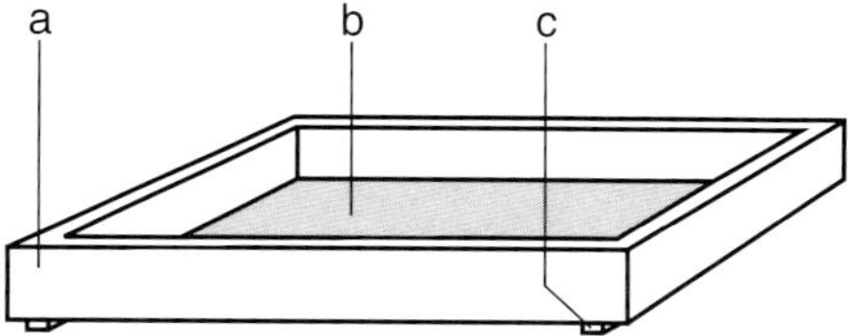

Fig. 38 Wooden frame for growing wheat germ. a) Wooden frame, b) wire mesh, c) feet.

small fan can help, if necessary. If the growing space gets little or no natural daylight, a fluorescent plant growing light must be used.

These lamps must be on for at least 5-6 hours every day. The wheat germ grows best at a temperature of 18-22°C.

If the wheat germ is grown in summer on a balcony or in the garden, it must be placed in the shade. When the weather is dry, the sprouts must be watered twice a day, but the roots must not be allowed to rot, because it makes the wheat germ unusable as food since the locusts also eat the roots. To feed wheat germ, it is removed from the tray, turned upside down, and portions are cut off with a sharp knife. Since the rooting is strong and entangled, it is almost impossible to pull it apart.

A different method for growing wheat germ can be used when less time is available or when 2-3 day absences are common, since it keeps the wheat moist longer. About 250 g of soaked wheat are mixed with about 21 pieces of large wood shavings, loosely filled into plastic bowls of about 10 x 10 x 5 cm and placed on a windowsill. They must be kept moist. Those who have a feel for watering can leave the bowls as they are, the rest of us should drill a few holes in the bottom and put the containers on top of small

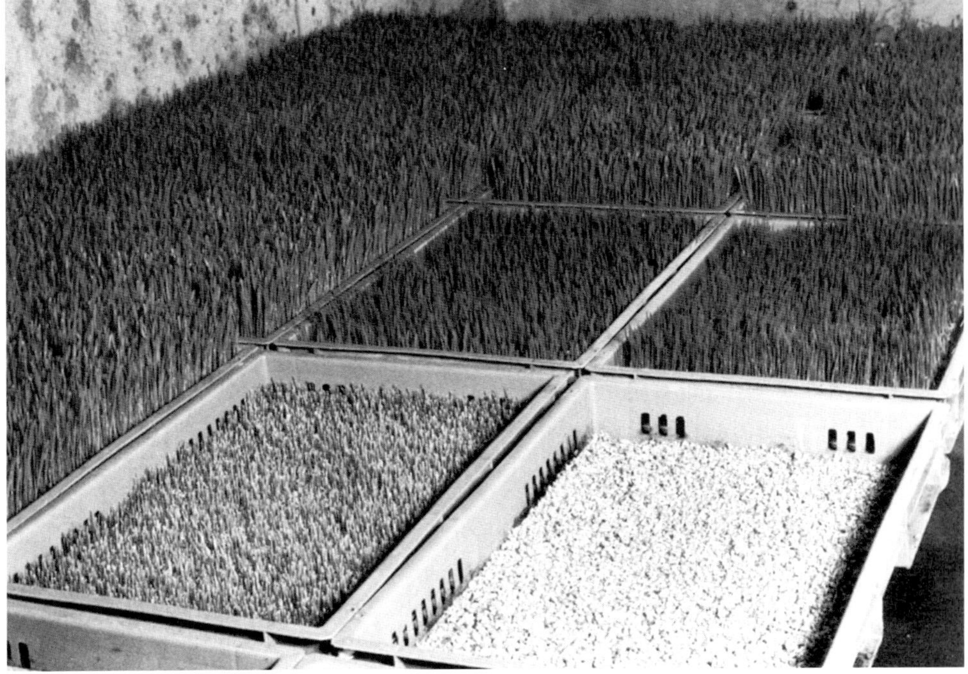

Fig. 39 Germinated wheat in various stages of development.

blocks in trays. The old rule still holds: too much water allows mold to grow.

Breeding Conditions:

Light and temperature: Migratory locusts are active during the day, and they love heat, so their setups require sufficient heat and light. With incandescent light bulbs or infrared heat emitters plus fluorescent bulbs, ideal conditions can be created in the breeding cages. The required wattages must be found by experimentation; for the home-built cage, an incandescent light bulb of 40-75 watts is enough. The preferred temperatures for each species are listed in the section on development times.

Locusts chew on heat tape, the tape will not deliver the required amounts of heat, and it would have to be installed in a false bottom for reasons of safety.

Humidity: If fresh food is offered, there is no need for drinking water. For *L. migratoria*, *S. gregaria* and *D. maroccanus* the air humidity is of no concern. *S. paranensis*, however, must be misted daily, as well as the larvae of all species until after their second molt.

The egg-laying substrate should always be evenly moist. Standing water must be avoided at all cost, as the eggs will rot. They tolerate a dry period of 4-6 days without problems, but embryo develop-ment will be delayed by 2-3 days. It takes quite a bit of practice to maintain the desired level of moisture.

Notes: We are often asked, how a locust breeding setup can actually be made to work. Those asking may have bought breeding pairs multiple times, but their breeding stock died after a short time even though they believe to have done everything right. One common mistake is that only adult animals are purchased which may have been fed exclusively on wheat germ, or lucerne and dandelion by their breeder. Private breeders mostly feed lettuce. This sudden change in diet after shipping, which already weakens the animals, is more than they can tolerate.

The following must be considered with newly acquired animals: They should be acclimatized gently, over the course of a day, to the preferred temperature and only be fed dry food. The next day they can be fed beech or oak leaves (in summer) and grated carrots (in winter) for fresh food. The dry food should not run out so that the animals can rebalance their hydration status. Only from the third day onwards should they be familiarized with lettuce and other foods. It is best to purchase larvae, of all stages, which can tolerate the change in environment much better. This also prevents production peaks in the setup.

Small-scale breeding setup: Breeding should be initiated with at least 10 breed-ing pairs and about 50 nymphs. The greens are placed on the floor of the cage and the dry food and grated carrots are offered in a shallow bowl. A freezer container is filled to the rim with substrate and placed in the cage in such a way that the females can get to it easily. It is recommended to keep two cages going, one for the breeding stock and one for the larvae. Once the females have busily buried eggs into the substrate and the first hatchings are expected in 1-2 days, the egg-laying container is moved to the second cage. The breeding animals receive a new egg-laying container.

After 14-20 days, when all the larvae have hatched from the first egg-laying container, it is removed and the substrate is thrown out. The container is washed and made ready for its next round.

It helps to attach a note to the cage with the various dates jotted down.

During molting the larvae are soft and vulnerable for 10-20 minutes and they fall easily prey to the cannibalistic desires of their cage mates. This makes it especially important that the cage for raising the larvae offer a large number of screen or other rough surfaces where the larvae can hang during their molt, and that enough fresh food is available to last until the next feeding.

The locusts receive fresh moist foods daily, and the old food must be removed; the dry food is inspected and replenished if necessary, at the latest after 3-4 days. For the rest of the time, it is best not to disturb the animals during breeding, egg laying, and molting.

Large-scale breeding: The care-taking process is the same for large setups as it is for small ones. However, the cages are considerably larger and offer room for 200-300 breeding pairs and about 1500 larvae until their third molt. For egg laying, 3-4 containers are placed in the cage. All containers that contain eggs are moved to a separate cage. Every 1-2 days, a new cage setup is started. In this way, the animals in each cage are of similar size, molt at almost the same time, and thus have no opportunity to eat their cage mates.

The following rule of thumb can be used: Of 100 locusts 70 can be harvested for food, 10 die, and the remaining 20 replenish the breeding stock.

To breed about 150,000 locusts in a year, 20 cages of 70 x 45 x 45 cm are required.

Poisoning, Diseases, and Pests: Since migrating locusts are very sensitive, poisonings must be mentioned: Residues of insecticides on fruit, lettuce, and vegetables are most certainly fatal. This is why store-bought fruit and vegetables must be washed thoroughly under running water; lettuce must be soaked for several hours with several water changes. Those who want to be on the safe side will keep a few "test subjects" in a separate container and the breeding stock only receives food that has been "tested." Many breeding setups have been destroyed by poisoned lettuce, and only a few eggs remained to save the breeding stock. Since large-scale breeders cannot take such a risk, they feed exclusively wheat germ. This is also recommended for noncommercial breeders who have the space to sprout wheat.

Locusts are often afflicted by a yeast fungus of the genus *Torulpsis*, which turns their abdomen coral-red to lilac. Reptiles that eat such locusts will have "blood" in their stool, which indicates large numbers of the yeast cells. This yeast is harmless to vivarium animals. In our experience this yeast spreads especially when the fresh food is too wet, or if apples and pears are the primary foods. Immediate raising of the temperature, a change in diet, and a little Nipagin (according to Prof. Frank) added to the dry food will prevent the worst. Locusts that have eaten Nipagin should not be used as food.

If the locusts are fed wild grasses, it should be expected that they will become infested with mermithid larvae, a nematode. They sit on grass leaves when the weather is moist and drill through the chitin exoskeleton of the locusts into their abdominal cavity when they get close. They grow inside the locusts and end up taking up all the space in the abdomen. Mermithids cause so-called parasitic castration, that is, the locust will not reach the imago stage and will not be able to reproduce. If many such nematodes are brought in, the breeding stock can die out within a few generations.

Mites are many a breeders' nightmare. If the show up in breeding cages, only one method promises relief: All the animals must be removed and the cage thoroughly cleaned with hot and soapy water. The surroundings of the cage should also be washed down. The locusts must be rinsed in a strainer with lukewarm water, and the egg-laying substrate must be destroyed, even if it contains eggs. Mites can gain a foothold primarily if food leftovers and feces are not removed, or if the setup is kept too moist.

Feeding: Since locusts do not hide but walk and jump around, they are especially suitable for chasing by vivarium animals. They can simply be tossed into terrariums, cages, or the water. Vivarium animals should be fed locusts in small amounts, since the surviving food animals eat the plants.

There is probably no other food animal that is accepted by so many different vivarium animals. Locusts can be offered to all insect eating animals including fish, amphibians, reptiles, birds, and mammals. For many species they make a good staple food. Prosimians and marmoset monkeys, for example, will go crazy chasing locusts. Praying mantises, bird spiders, and scorpions will not refuse locusts either, and for many plant-eating animals, like spiny-tailed lizards, they make a welcome supplement.

Advantages and Disadvantages:

Advantages:

- High-quality, fiber-rich food for all insect-eating vivarium animals
- Setups can be kept in living spaces without risk
- Medium amount of work, but daily feeding is required
- Low-cost if fed wheat germ
- Almost free of smell

  Disadvantages:
- Sensitive people are bothered by the chirping of courting males
- Daily inspection necessary
- Cultivating wheat grass takes up much space
- Fruit, vegetables, and lettuce as food are expensive in winter

Indian Stick Insect (*Carausius morosus*) Annam Stick Insect (*Baculum extradentatum*)

Carausius morosus (Fig. 40): As the common name indicates, these insects are stick-shaped. Adults reach a body length of up to 80 mm at a diameter of about 5 mm. When they rest, their long, thin legs are held tightly next to the body, the front pair reaching above the head together with the antennae for a length of up to 30 mm and more. Their green color camouflages the stick insects between the leaves, only the red inside of their thighs forms a contrast. Only one male occurs for over 1000 females. This is why mostly female *Carausius morosus* are known, which will

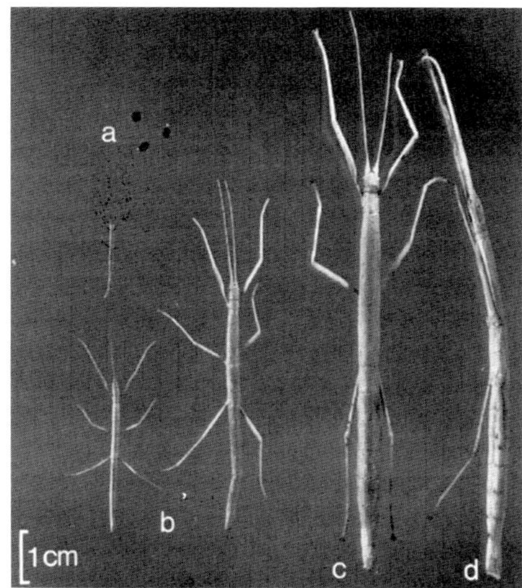

Fig. 40 Indian stick insect (*Carausius morosus*). a) Eggs, b) larvae, c) female from above, d) female lateral view.

reproduce pathogenetically for many generations; that is, their unfertilized eggs will develop into fully functional animals. The brown eggs (Fig. 42b) are ovaloid, 2 mm thick and 2.5 mm long; from them hatch 13 mm long, barely 1 mm in diameter, brown-green larvae that turn green after their first molt.

Baculum extradentatum (Fig. 41): This species has known males and females. The females lay both fertilized and unfertilized eggs after mating; larvae hatch from about 60% of the eggs (facultative parthenogenesis). The difference in size between the genders is considerable: while the males grow only to 65-70 mm long with a 1.5-2 mm diameter, the females are even larger than the Indian stick insects, namely 85-95 mm at a diameter of 4-4.5 mm. The antennae are only about 20 mm long. The front legs appear excessively long at 70-75

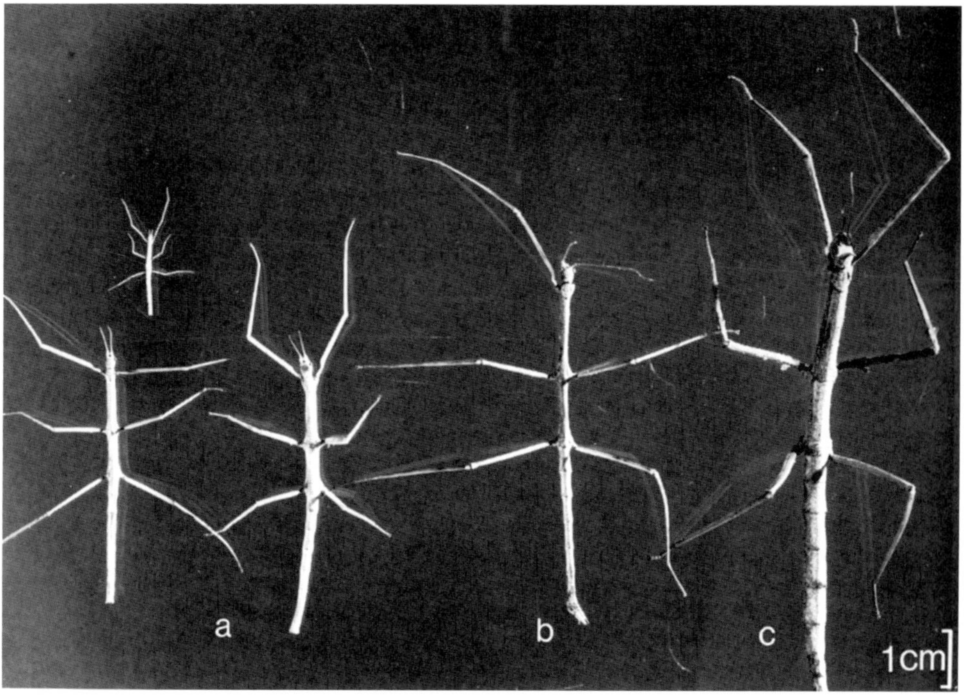

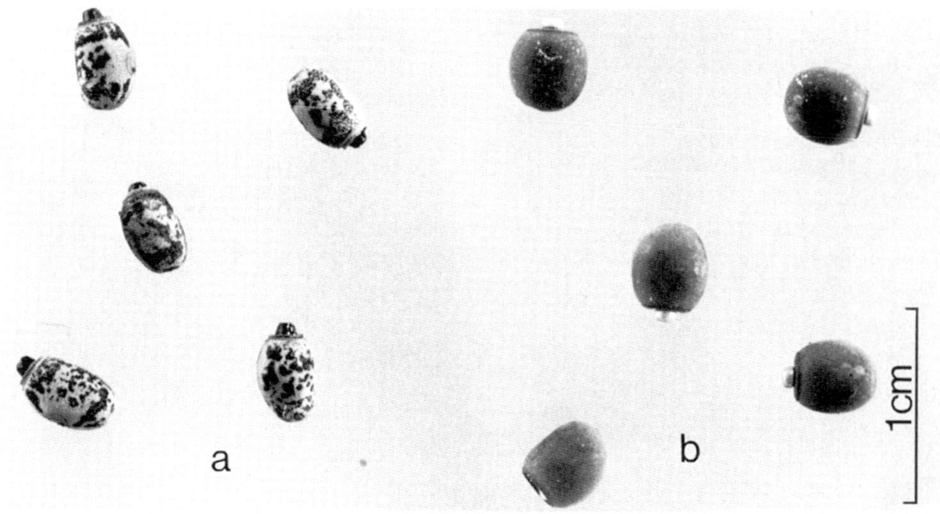

Fig. 41 Annam stick insect *(Baculum extradentatum)*. a) larvae, b) male, c) female.

Fig. 42 a) Eggs Annam stick insect, b) eggs of Indian stick insect.

mm. Adults animals show a gray-brown coloring; they legs have a reddish tinge; the medium-sized larvae are light brown. The edges of almost all leg segments are covered with fine thorns, as are the bodies of the females. Larvae of medium size, 30-40 mm, already reveal their gender: The females and their larvae have an impressive thorn above their eyes, which can reach 1 mm in length in adult animals. In addition, a leaf-like enlarged thorn points backwards from the thigh of the middle pair of legs; each lower leg also has two larger thorns. The male larvae have light-green thighs on their rear legs.

They gray-black mottled(Fig. 42 a) eggs are 3 mm long and 2 mm wide and larger than those of *Carausius morosus*. The hatchlings measure about 12 mm and 1 mm diameter and have an olive-green body with dark leg joints and light green extremities.

Development Times: *Carausius morosus*: An adult stick insect lays 1-2 eggs every night during her 6 to maximum 12-month life if fed well, a total of 200-450 eggs. The hatch rate is 80-90%. At 22-24°C the young hatch after 13-20 weeks. After 5-6 molts they are adults, which is after 4-5 months at a temperature of 19-22°C.

Baculum extradentatum: This species develops much faster. At 25-26°C the eggs hatch in our experience after 3-4 weeks. Bergegard (1958) lists an incubation time of 6 weeks for fertilized and 8 weeks for unfertilized eggs at 27°C. At 18°C they require, according to the same author, 7 months to develop. The animals reach adulthood in about 10 weeks at a tempera-ture of 25-26°C. The lifespan for adults is 3-5 months.

Containers, Substrate, and Equipment: Larger Plexiglas or glass aquariums make suitable containers for stick insects. The lid can be made from a wooden frame covered with screen. The insides of the sides of the aquarium can be covered with curtain fabric or screen so that the animals have more places to climb. This is especially important if the cage is to contain larvae, which need more space for molting.

In a home-built cage (see Figs. 43 & 44), all the inner sides, and the top are covered with screen. If the door is made from glass, the interior can be better observed. Absorbent paper like newspaper or kitchen paper towels can be used as the substrate; if the cage has a false bottom of wire mesh and a drawer, no substrate is required.

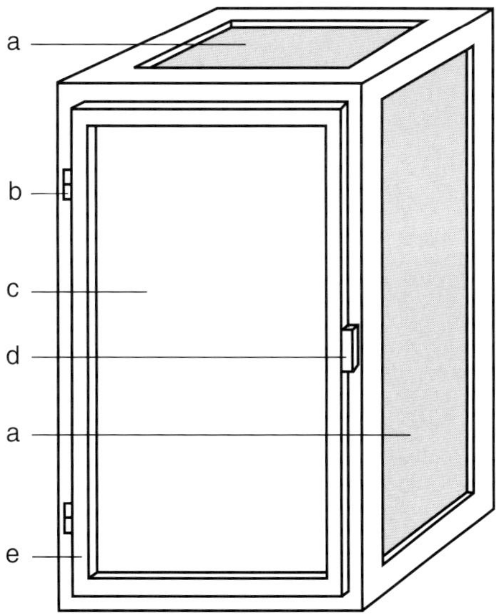

Fig. 43 Home-built wooden cage for stick insects (40 x 40 x 70 cm). a) Screen, b) hinge, c) glass panel or screen, d) lock, e) door.

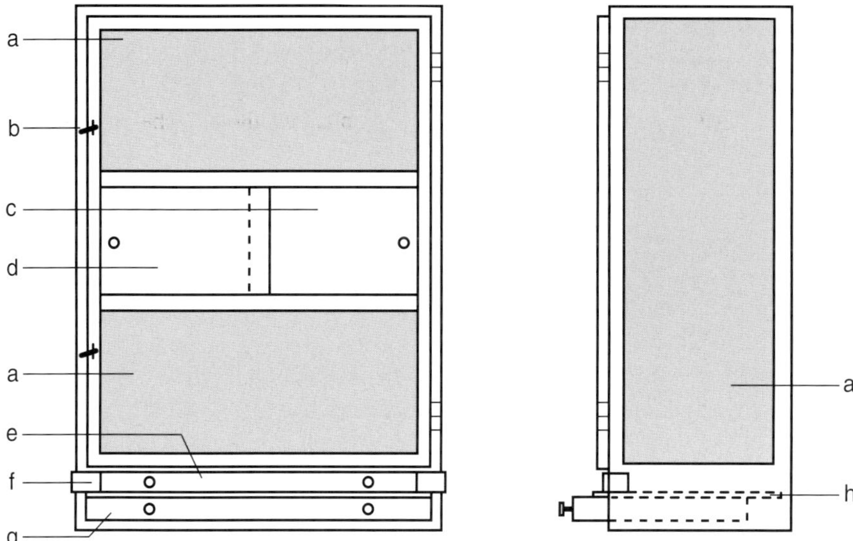

Fig. 44 Wooden cage for stick insects; front and side view. a) Screen, b) lock, c) and d) sliding glass panels, e) sliding panel, f) guiding rail, g) drawer, h) removable false bottom.

The branches that the stick insects should eat should be put in a vase so that they stay fresh longer. Stick insects drink little. Use a wide, low, but narrow-necked bottle or a low glass with a lid in which several holes of 5-10 mm have been drilled. The branches are fitted through these holes. To refill water, simply put a hose or pipe through the hole in the bottle or lid.

Food: *Carausius morosus* eats all sorts of leaves. In summer there are no problems; branches of—unsprayed!—fruit trees, linden tree, hazel, chestnut, or beech, are eaten as much as rose, raspberry, or blackberry leaves. In winter, ivy and blackberry can be fed. Do not feed ivy to animals that are to be used as food. To grow Tradescantias as is sometimes recommended only makes sense for a small number of animals, otherwise there are too many plants that must be cared for. These plants should not be fed to the stick insects a few days before they are to be used as food if the vivarium animals show a distaste for the tannic acid flavor. *Baculum extradentatum* is fed on blackberry leaves all year and in summer also on raspberry leaves, and branches from beeches, oaks, linden and other leafy trees. Ivy, lilac, laburnum, laurel, and elder are poisonous to stick insects.

In winter you can fall back on the leaves of the evergreen oak *Quercus* x *turneri pseudoturneri*, an oak that only sheds its leaves just before the new ones emerge.

Breeding Conditions:

Light: Stick insects are content with a poorly lighted space. They should be exposed to a day-night cycle.

Temperature: Stick insects thrive well at room temperature (18-22°C); for breeding the temperature should not fall below

102

18°C. At 28°C they are most prolific, and at 7-8°C reproduction ceases. Depending on the desired reproductive rate, the setups can be kept warmer or cooler.

Humidity: If fresh leaves are always available, their moisture is enough for *Carausius morosus*. It is better, though, to mist the containers once a day. For the Annam stick insect this is mandatory, since they need to drink. Too much moisture on the bottom should be avoided so that the feces do not start to mold.

Notes: Since for stick insects the differences between larger and smaller setups are only in scale, the following notes apply to both.

Stick insects are active at night. Therefore, their cage should be cleaned during the day, otherwise the insects are hard to control. If an aquarium that is opened from the top is used, it makes the job much easier if the animals can be moved to another container; it is advantageous to always have a spare setup ready for this purpose.

For young animals until their last molt, a long cage with a length-to-width ratio of 2:1 works well, with a double-door and a wire-mesh floor. One half of the cage holds the older branches; when they are eaten, a new glass with branches is put in the other half. A few days later, the remaining animals can be shaken or picked from the bare branches; the stick insects use their claws to hold tightly to their branches so that some patience may be required to pry them loose, especially if you need to transfer several hundred or thousand animals!

The feces fall through the wire mesh, collect in the drawer, and are easy to remove. The calmer adults can easily be kept in such containers.

To make better use of the available space in ontainers with adult animals, it is better to replace all the branches at every cleaning.

The eggs of these two species develop also when they rest on a dry substrate. Therefore, they need not be separated from the droppings. If you wish to do this anyway, you can sift the eggs of *Carausius morosus* with an ordinary wire screen. However, when ivy leaves are fed, the droppings can be so large, they will also remain in the sieve.

The more-frequently described method of separating the eggs from the feces by floating them in water and scooping them off is less ideal, since too many eggs remain on the bottom.

Pests and Diseases: Certainly, stick insects can harbor parasites, but we do not know of any that affect their breeding.

Feeding: When feeding stick insects it must be considered that any stick insects that remain in the a terrarium overnight will chew on the terrarium plants, then sit so quietly and hidden the next day that the terrarium inhabitants most likely will not notice them. Therefore, stick insects should be offered to your animals by hand. This is different for nocturnal vivarium animals; but they will not always eat up all the available food either.

Because of their unwieldy shape and their nocturnal lifestyle, stick insects are not overly favored. Consider them an easy to breed supplemental food that is offered to small and medium-sized lizards and amphibians. Especially arboreal reptiles like chameleons, several geckos, agamas, and iguanas appreciate them for variety in their diet.

Advantages:
- Can be bred at room temperature in a moderately bright location
- Do not need daily attention—except for misting of *B. extradentatum*—only after leaves have been consumed

Disadvantages
- Transferring animals is tedious
- Suitable food for relatively few vivarium animals

Beetles (Coleoptera)

About 300,000 beetle species form the largest insect order Coleoptera. Its members include tiny and gigantic animals, and beetles that inhabit the most diverse environments with greatly varying dietary preferences. In spite of this, a beetle is recognized instantly. Only the larvae, which often hide in the ground, rotting wood, or manure are a less familiar sight. Beetles usually have a stocky build. The shape of their body is primarily influenced by the first large thoracic segment and the hardened forewings (elytra) that form a protective cover. The front of the chest sometimes carries grotesquely shaped growths, as for example, seen on the rhinoceros beetles. The hardened forewings protect the delicate rear wings und the whole abdomen. The head is usually small; it can also be decorated with eye-catching appendages, as for example, gigantic mouth parts (stag beetle) or horns (goliath beetle). Head, thorax, and elytra are often of the same color in a matching pattern. The best-known food animal, the yellow mealworm beetle and its larvae, the mealworms, and several other beetles that are used as food animals, belong to the family of the darkling beetles (Tenebrionidae). The smallest beetle discussed here belongs to the family of the seed weevils (Bruchidae). From the family of the dung beetles (Scarabaeidae) and the subfamily of the flower beetles (Cetoninae) we introduce a member who is not only for its value as food but also because of its beauty.

Lesser Mealworm Beetle (*Alphitobius diaperinus*)

Description: The body of the shiny brown and black lesser mealworm beetle (Fig. 45) is egg-shaped and hairless. The scutellum is widest at its base and curves and narrows towards the front. The elytra show fine, dot-like indentations that are arranged lengthwise. The beetles reach a size of 5.5-6.5 mm and a width of 3-3.5 mm. From the longish, milky-white eggs of 0.6 mm length hatch 0.8-1 mm long larvae that can get up to 13 mm long and 2 mm in diameter. They are soft-skinned, light brown with darker bands, and move swiftly. Breeding stock with lighter larvae can also be found. In the English- and Dutch-speaking areas the term "buffalo worms" is often used. The light-yellow pupae measure 5-6 mm.

This beetle is mostly known under the wrong designation *Alphitobius ovatus. A. ovatus* is an old name for another *Alphitobius* species, *A. laevigatus*, which is rarer and probably rarely bred. With a size 4.5-5 mm, it also remains smaller than *A. diaperinus* and its color is dull black-brown. Another difference is that the scutellum is at its widest in the middle in this species.

Development Times: Few food animals develop as fast as the lesser mealworm beetle. At a temperature of 23-25°C the

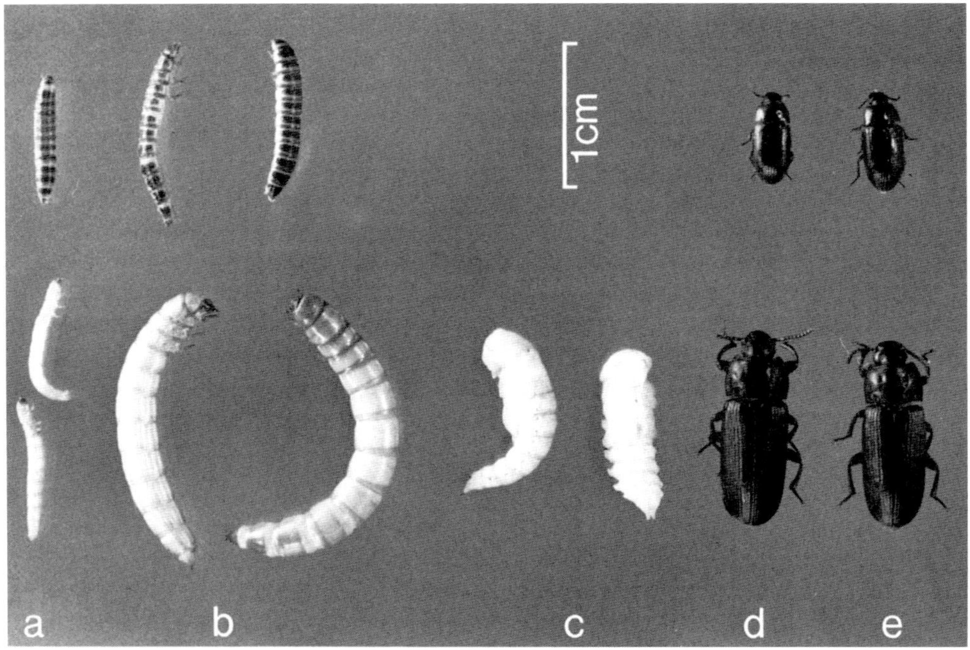

Fig. 45 Top: Lesser mealworm beetle *(Alphitobius diaperinus)*. Bottom: Yellow mealworm beetle *(Tenebrio molitor)*. a) Small larvae, b) fully grown larvae, c) pupae, d) males, e) females.

development time is only 7-8½ weeks, at 27-28°C only 5½-6½ weeks. If the temperature is raised to 30°C, the time is reduced to 4-5 weeks. A range of 27-28°C has been shown to be the best breeding temperature; the females are not quite as prolific, but if the reproductive rate is higher, cannibalism becomes a limiting factor. The minimum temperature for a breeding setup is 20°C.

In a well-stocked container of larvae, the temperature will rise by a few degrees because of the heat produced by the larvae. At the optimal temperature the larvae hatch after 4-6 days; they pupate after 23-27 days. The pupae rest for 5 days. The first matings occur 2 days after the beetles hatch; 2-4 days later the females lay the first eggs, in clumps of 8-15 eggs. The life span of this beetle is around 6 months. A female produces up to 1000 eggs during this time.

Container, Substrate, and Equipment: Small-to medium-sized containers with smooth sides and a lid that is covered with screen or gauze for ventilation are well suited, like large cans, freezer boxes, plastic aquariums, plastic tubs, and similar containers. The containers for the larvae should be at least 8 cm high, the containers for the breeding beetles 15 cm. For large-scale breeding plastic boxes as they are used for breeding rats or mice are practical because they can be stored in racks.

Lesser mealworms live like kings: Their substrate should consist of dry food, for example, a mixture of oats, egg-laying mash for chickens, and bran. This mixture is sprinkled in the container in a thin layer, then covered with several layers of egg cartons or corrugated cardboard for the beetles, and corrugated cardboard and paper for the larvae.

The beetles like to lay their eggs on moist pieces of fabric.

Since the setups thrive in the dark and at higher temperatures, they can be placed in a heated cabinet as described on page 22. Infrared heat emitters or heating pads can also be used. A heated room to store the setups is ideal, for example, the boiler room in winter.

Food: Lesser mealworm beetles are omnivores. They can be fed on an exclusively vegetarian diet, but the best results occur only when animal proteins are also fed.

Like for many breeding setups, a separation of dry from moist foods has proven useful. Bran should not be the only dry food, but it should be mixed with oats, dog flakes, and chicken mash. In addition, feed wheat germ, chicken feed, and a variety of pellet foods, as well as dry meat or fish occasionally.

For moist food, the beetles receive grated carrots, potato slices, apple slices, banana, greens, and softened white bread. They like to eat beef fat that is cut into strips and allowed to dry a little before it is fed. The best breeding results have been documented when the animals get the following super mix as a supplement: 200 g laying-hen mash, 100 g oats, 100 g soy meal, 100 g milk powder, 250 g old, crumbled white bread and 50 g dry or brewers yeast, all mixed together. Small portions are moistened with enough water to form a thick dough that can be shaped into patties. These are placed on top of the dry food. For the beetles the food is meted out in portions that are completely eaten within 3-4 hours; otherwise the females will deposit their eggs into the patties, which arc then eaten. These beetles require a lot of moist food.

Breeding Conditions:

Light: Lesser mealworm beetles are shy of light and are happy in a dark spot. Breeding seems to work better if they are kept without light.

Temperature: The optimal breeding temperature is around 27-28°C. Below 20°C reproduction ceases; at about 30 °C cannibalism increases.

Humidity: The relative air humidity can be low, 30-50% is enough. The animals must have moist foods available at all times.

Notes:

Small-scale breeding: For a small breeding setup at least 2 containers should be used, if possible, so that the beetles and their larvae can be kept separately. If the beetles are not fed moist food every day, they will eat the freshly molted larvae and pupae and cause major losses. If dead black larvae and pupae are found in the container, it is a sign of trouble!

For the beetles, a small container of 30 x 20 x 15 cm is big enough; the larvae can be raised in a tub with a footprint of 40 x 30 cm.

If the collected larvae are moved into a separate container every week, 5 smaller containers are all that is needed. It is best to keep larvae of the same size in each container.

About 200 beetles make for a good initial

breeding stock. They are used to carefully increase the stock. The following example assumes a development time of about 6 weeks at about 27-28°C, and one tub each for beetles and larvae.

The beetles are placed in their prepared container and are fed daily with small amounts of moist food. *A. diaperinus* is rather tolerant of moldy food, but it is still recommended to keep the setup relatively free of mold. Therefore, leftover moist food should be removed twice a week. The fabric pieces for egg laying are kept just moist enough that the food underneath does not become moldy.

After 2 weeks, the eggs and small larvae are for the first time separated from the beetles. First the egg cartons or the corrugated cardboard and the fabric pieces are gently shaken out and moved into a separate container. Then all of the substrate is strained through a sieve with a mesh size of 1.5 mm. Beetles and larger pieces of dry food are returned into the breeding container, as well as the other "furniture," after the dry food has been replenished. The strained out substrate contains the eggs and young larvae, and it is put into the second, larger container, which is also filled with substrate and supplied with fresh food every day.

After another 2 weeks, the substrate from the container with the breeding beetles is strained again and the eggs and larvae are transferred to the second container. There the first larvae have in the meantime grown up and are ready to pupate. A small number of larvae may have already been harvested for food. The larvae like to crawl between layers of newspaper or fabric and can easily be harvested there. Of course, a supply of breeding beetles

must always be retained. A number of adult larvae are placed in a shallow container that is lined with newspaper. Until they pupate, they receive small amounts of moist food. Alternatively, you can wait a few days longer and remove the pupae from the larvae container. The pupae must absolutely be undisturbed, otherwise the beetles hatch deformed. The newly emerged beetles like to hide in a small rag, which can then be shaken out into the breeding container.

Every 4-6 weeks—before new larvae are added—the larvae should be separated from their feces. A sieve with a mesh-size of about 0.5 mm is good for this purpose. Depending on the requirements and the temperature, a certain routine can be established and used to decide on the number and sizes of containers.

The amount of substrate is determined according to the following rule of thumb: To raise 500 g of larvae, 300 g of food substrate are required. One hundred fully grown larvae weigh 2.5 g.

The lesser mealworm beetle is considered a pest and is not welcome in warehouses that are used for food storage. We must prevent it from getting into our own food supplies. It is therefore extremely important that the breeding container have a tight-fitting lid so that the beetles cannot fly off. This beetle should also not be tolerated in other breeding setups, for example, mealworms or crickets, as it will eat their eggs and larvae. If it gets into the crickets, it can be carefully picked out; a simple method to remove it from a mealworm setup is described on page 113.

Large-scale breeding: The methods for the large-scale setups are similar to those for small-scale breeding. If the substrate is strained into a new container every 2-3 days, this guarantees even growth for the larvae. The number and size of the containers depends on the desired amounts of animals.

Storage: If they are mixed with at least an equal volume of bran, the larvae can be stored for up to 4 weeks; the temperature should not fall below 15°C and not rise above 20°C.

Pests and Diseases: Another advantage of breeding these beetles is that, to our knowledge, they are not afflicted by diseases or pests. Even mites, which can occur in all setups, do not become established in these setups. Maybe the beetles eat the mites? However, in very small setups with few beetles, we have observed some mites.

Feeding: The simplest and easiest method is to offer the beetles and larvae in a bowl with smooth sides. Only for fish, small numbers are sprinkled on the water surface. To remove larvae from their setup with the least work, take advantage of their preference for crawling on top of the substrate. Bury a can into the substrate so that its rim is even with the substrate surface (see also Helbig, 1985). A rectangular dish that is adjacent to the side is ideal. Overnight, plenty of larvae will fall into the dish.

Small frogs, toads, lizards, birds, and invertebrates especially love the lesser mealworm larvae. They are also suitable for raising the young of larger vivarium animals. Birds like the lightly colored larvae in particular. Since the larvae are soft-skinned, they can be fed in large numbers without fear of damage to the vivarium animals. The beetles, however, are so hard, that few animals can eat them.

Damage and losses can occur if the larvae escape inside the cages and vivariums since they will eat reptile eggs and will damage nestlings, especially those of ground breeders; the larvae will also crawl along wooden sides and branches, if possible, into nesting boxes.

Advantages and Disadvantages:

Advantages:

- Short development time
- High reproductive rate
- Easy to digest and, if fed well, high-quality animal food
- Requires little space compared to yield

Disadvantages:

- Setups require daily attention
- Smells if too much fresh food is offered
- Can cause damage in vivariums and bird cages
- Pest in food supplies

Yellow Mealworm Beetle (*Tenebrio molitor*)

Description: The shiny body of the 15-18 mm long, about 5 mm wide and 3.5 mm tall mealworm beetle (Fig. 45) is black brown to black on top and red brown on the underside. The elytra show small, point-like indentations that are arranged in rows. The genders can only be distinguished with much practice. The tibiae of the front legs of the males are curved, those of the females are straight. The antennae are about 3.5 mm long.

From the 1.3-1.6 mm long whitish, slender eggs hatch dirt-yellow larvae of 1.6-2 mm size that become a darker color after 12-14 days. After 9-12 molts, the larvae reach a size of 25-28 mm and a diameter of 2.5-3.5

mm. The corn-yellow larvae, commonly called mealworms, can in exceptional cases get up to 34 mm long. The pupa is usually as long as the beetle that emerges from it. The beetles are first whitish and soft, and their exoskeleton hardens only after 1-2 days.

Development Times: The development times of the mealworm beetle depend on the temperature and the amounts of food that are available. At 27°C and with optimal nutrition the generations follow each other about every 10-12 weeks. The beetles reach sexual maturity after 10-12 days; 8 days after mating egg laying starts. The eggs hatch after 5-7 days, the larvae develop in 6-7 weeks, and the pupae rest for another 6-10 days. The larvae only grow fast in the last 2 weeks; 4 week-old larvae measure 1.5 cm. At temperatures of 23-25°C the total development time becomes 3½ to 4 months, at 20-21°C about 5 months.

Under favorable conditions, the beetles live for about 3 months. The females lay 160 eggs.

Containers, Substrate, and Equipment: Mealworm beetles used to be raised in wooden boxes because they hold their temperature well. However, the larvae would eat through the wood and the boxes needed to be replaced frequently. Today, plastic aquariums, larger multipurpose tubs, or PVC tubs are used.

For large-scale breeding, the same plastic trays that are used for mice and rats are also used. The sides of the breeding container should be at least 15 cm high. For smaller setups, containers of 5 l volume are big enough to raise 500-800 g of mealworms. The container for the breeding stock must be covered with a screen cover so that the beetles cannot escape. Mealworms cannot climb smooth walls so that their container can remain uncovered. The substrate, like that for the lesser mealworm beetles, consists of the dry food itself, which is filled in to a height of several centimeters. The beetles like to crawl underneath paper or a layer of egg cartons. To harvest mealworms, place a few moistened rags or layers of paper into the container a few hours before the larvae are needed. The larvae can then be found and removed without any need for digging around in the whole container. Since the females drop their eggs any-where they please, no special egg-laying substrate is required.

To house a small-scale breeding setup, a home-built climate-controlled cabinet is especially suitable (see page 23). In it, the humidity can easily be kept at the desirable level of 70%. The temperature is adjusted depending on the desired development time.

For large-scale efforts, a climate-controlled room should be available.

Food: How the mealworms are fed determines not only the speed and quality of their development but also their value as food animals. The mealworm often has a bad reputation as a food animal, because its quality leaves much to be desired when it is raised on low-quality foods. On bran alone, no valuable mealworms can be raised!

We have had good results with the following food mixtures:

Mixture A:

    250 g wheat flour
    250 g oats
    100 g laying hen mash
    350 g wheat bran

Mixture B:

- 250 g wheat flour
- 250 g oats
- 100 g soy meal
- 70 g cornmeal
- 30 g dry or brewer's yeast
- 300 g wheat bran

Between those two mixtures, differences in weight are evident. Mealworms that were fed with mixture A weighed 42-48 mg, those with on mixture B 54-66 mg! A development time of 6-7 weeks for the larvae could only be reached feeding mixture B; those larvae fed with mixture A needed 2 extra weeks. If mixture A is to be used, adding yeast is highly recommended. These dry-food mixtures serve also as the substrate in which the mealworms and their beetles live. The amounts required depend on the number of breeding beetles (see Notes). For variety, dry dog or cat food, dried bread, crackers, semolina, and ground rice can be offered.

The fresh food consists primarily of carrot and apple slices that are placed with the cut surface on top of the substrate, but also dandelion leaves and other greens. Fresh meat should be offered sparingly as a supplemental food because it spoils quickly and smells bad.

Breeding Conditions:

Light: The mealworm beetle and its larvae have an aversion to light so that the setups can be placed in complete darkness.

Temperature: Optimal development occurs around 27-28°C. Temperatures above 40°C are deadly for the beetles and the larvae, but even at 35°C the rate of reproduction is reduced; only 30-40% of the eggs hatch compared to 70% at the lower temperatures.

A large number of larvae produce quite a bit of heat, which must be taken into account. The minimum temperature for a breeding setup is 19°C.

Humidity: The weight of the larvae does not only depend on the temperature but also significantly on the air humidity in which they are raised. In experiments by Martin, Rivers, and Cowgill (1976), the larvae that were kept at 21°C weighed in average after 12 weeks:

- 18 mg at 30% relative air humidity
- 38 mg at 50% relative air humidity
- 68 mg at 70% relative air humidity

We repeated this experiment at 27°C and 6 weeks development time and measured the following:

- 32 mg at 30% relative air humidity
- 41 mg at 50% relative air humidity
- 66 mg at 70% relative air humidity

Do not be tempted to keep the mealworms at higher levels of humidity as this will inevitably lead to mold in the substrate, which damages the larvae.

Even when the beetles are kept at a humidity level of 60-70%, they must still be fed regularly with moist food, which also satisfies their water requirements. Without fresh food the beetles will survive for 4-6 days, and the development of the larvae is much slower and mortality is high.

If there is a lack of fresh food, or too many animals are in the container, newly molted larvae and pupae will be chewed on, and they will die and turn black.

Notes: The question all vivarium enthusiasts have to ask is when it might be worth the trouble to breed their own mealworms since they can be bought at pet stores and ordered from breeders. This is certainly also a question of time and money. We think that the efforts to breed are worthwhile only if more than 100 g of larvae per week are needed. Those who wish to make a living of breeding mealworms must produce and sell at least 10-20 kg per week.

Small-scale breeding: If you only need a small number of mealworms but would like to raise your own anyway, you can make do with one box.

This also makes the bothersome sifting unnecessary and the larvae can be harvested by baiting them with moist food. After a few weeks, a new container is set up and stocked with beetles, while the first container is kept until the last mealworm has been removed. Especially for people with asthma, this is the preferred method.

For a setup from which 100-200 g of larvae can be harvested weekly six containers measuring 30 x 20 x 15 cm are needed: one for the breeding beetles, one for larvae for food, three for raising larvae, and one as a spare.

We start with 300 g of larvae. All the beetles, about 1200 of them, become our breeding stock. We fill their container with 300 g of substrate, that is, dry food mixture, a little bit of moist food, and several layers of paper on top; then the container is stocked and the lid fastened. The rest of the process is similar to the one for the lesser mealworm beetles. To make sure that the beetles can breed undisturbed, they are separated from the substrate, which contains eggs and small larvae, at certain times. If the mealworm beetles are kept at 27°C, they are sorted out every 5 weeks; the beetles and the substrate are emptied into a sieve with a 4 mm mesh-size, and the substrate is sifted into a second container. The beetles are returned to their original container on a layer of fresh substrate. This procedure is repeated every 2 weeks. The substrate is sifted into a new container every time, until after 11 weeks all five containers are filled. Now larvae from the first container should be large enough to be used as food.

At the same time, it is also necessary to separate them from their feces by using a 0.6 mm mesh-size sieve and to renew their dry food supply.

Two weeks later the larvae in the next container are sifted and added to the tub with the largest larvae; in this manner, there are always mealworms available for feeding. To save on the 6th container, you can wash out the container that was emptied and use it for sifting the beetles. Every 14 days about 1/6 of the larvae that are ready to pupate are separated out to guarantee a steady supply of breeding stock for a continuously producing setup. These chores repeat without breaks. It takes a bit of practice until the desired amounts of mealworms can be raised reliably.

People who suffer from asthma or allergies should only sift the substrate wearing a dust mask and preferably do it outdoors; the fine dust heavily irritates the respiratory tracts.

This setup can, of course, be scaled as desired. The use of 6-8 larger containers in which up to 800 g of larvae can be raised per week seems especially workable. This requires about 3000 beetles for breeding stock. The procedures are the same; however, eggs and young larvae are sifted out weekly and put into a fresh container each time.

In a three-part report Siegfried Kirschke (1985) describes his practical method for harvesting 150-200 g larvae weekly in a setup that he has developed over the last 10 years after experimenting for 20 years. In his experience uniform heat from below, wheat bran plus carrots (dandelion sprouts in spring) for food, and several layers of fabric on top are the most important factors. Details and procedures can found in his report.

Large-scale breeding: Two factors are important for a large-scale setup: constant temperature and precise procedures. The procedures for large and small-scale setups are similar. However, now thousands of breeding beetles are housed in large containers. The substrate must be sifted and the larvae distributed into several tubs at least once a week. If necessary, the medium-sized larvae are separated from their droppings and placed into as much new substrate as they need until they pupate, are harvested, or are sold. A specialized sifter with a catch tray (Fig. 46) makes this job much easier.

The breeding stock must be constantly observed and dead beetles replaced. When working at this large a scale pupae and beetles cannot be picked out by hand anymore, so additional containers are required for large larvae and for pupae. Beetles that hatch from their pupae are defenseless and are often eaten by the larvae, which makes them useless for breeding.

Larvae that are ready to pupate are placed into a container with substrate and are fed more carrots. Once some of these meal-worms have pupated, all of the substrate is dumped into a 4 mm sieve, put on top of the container, shaken a little, and left there until the larvae have crawled out through the mesh. Light from above accelerates this

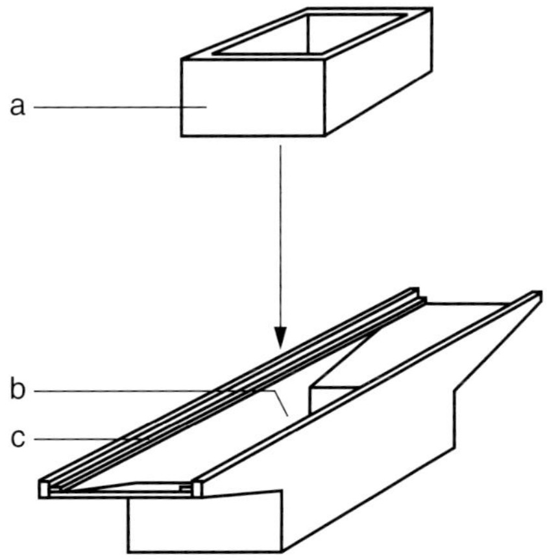

Fig. 46 Sieve and collecting tray with guide rails made of PVC or wood; for sifting larvae of yellow mealworm beetle, lesser mealworm beetle, and fly maggots. a) Sieve with exchangeable screen inserts of varying mesh sizes, b) catch tray, c) guide rail for sieve.

procedure. The pupae, which remain in the sieve, are distributed into a tub that is filled to 2 cm with bran and covered with 1-2 layers of egg cartons. The beetles can hatch undisturbed and usually crawl onto the egg cartons from where they can easily be transferred into the breeding container.

Storage: At 8°C mealworms can be stored for 2 months and more. At least as much bran as larvae must be mixed by volume.

Pests and Diseases: Well-known parasites of mealworms are gregarines, which live in the intestine of the larvae. Gregarines are single-celled organisms of the class Apicomplexa (previously: Sporozoa). As mentioned in the section on cockroaches, it has been determined that gregarines are not harmful to either their host or the vivarium animals that eat the mealworms.

Especially large breeding setups can get

infested with *Necrobia rufipes*, the red-legged ham beetle. This is a 6 mm long, metallic green, shiny beetle that eats the eggs and small larvae of the mealworm beetle. It can only be controlled by persistently picking the beetles out by hand; with much patience, it can be exterminated in that manner.

The lesser mealworm beetle can become a pest; it loves to nibble on pupae and freshly molted larvae. With a little bit of patience it can be exterminated in the following manner: A smooth-sided bowl that has to be as tall as the substrate is deep, is placed into the mealworm tub so that its edge is at the same level as the top of the substrate. It is emptied twice daily; almost exclusively larvae of the lesser mealworm beetle fall into it.

If the mealworms are raised at their preferred air humidity of 60-70%, mites are practically unavoidable. They can be controlled in two ways: One is that the beetles, pupae, and larvae are thoroughly rinsed in a sieve under warm water and all the equipment is thoroughly cleaned. However, this means the loss of all smaller larvae. Alternatively, the air humidity is temporarily reduced to 30%, no moist food is fed, and the mites are baited with moist woolen rags that are placed in the containers. Two to three times a day the rags are gently removed and the mites killed by running boiling water over the rags.

Feeding: Mealworms and their beetles cannot escape from bowls with smooth sides, therefore they can often be often in this way. With tweezers, they have to be pinched tightly, so the needle is more suitable.

Birds will sometimes tear apart the mealworms, and sometimes they cannot digest the wiry larvae. Ideally, they are only fed newly molted, soft mealworms. This is only possible if the mealworms are home bred, since store-bought mealworms are already past their last molt.

For many vivarium animals, mealworms are the primary food item. Therefore, they have been nutritionally analyzed, and it has been found that they do not consist just of fat, which is commonly asserted; about 13% of their live mass is fat, and 23% is protein. Nevertheless, their fat content is high enough, that they should not be fed as the sole food. Mealworms contain calcium and phosphorus at a ratio of 1:3 to 1:14 depending on their diet. Since vertebrates require calcium and phosphorus at a ratio of 1.2:1 to 1.5:1 for healthy bone structure, calcium must be supplemented, either directly or via the mealworms. Experiments by Zwart and Rulkens (1979) showed that mealworms that are kept on nothing but Carnicon for 24 hours acquire a healthy Ca:Ph ratio of 1.38:1. Carnicon is a multivitamin/mineral preparation with a Ca/P-ratio of 20:1; it is produced by the Trouw Company in Putten in the Netherlands. Mealworms will not consume pure calcium carbonate.

Not for no reason is the mealworm the best-known food animal for insect eaters: most species accept it happily. The pupae and beetles are also appreciated by many animals, as for example, insect-eating birds, frogs and toads, lizards, turtles, and predatory invertebrates, such as praying mantises, predatory bugs, and ground-dwelling spiders.

In addition, a significant number of medium-sized mammals also like mealworms, as for example, elephant shrews, marmoset monkeys, and pottos.

Advantages and Disadvantages:

Advantages:
- Requires little space for small-scale operation
- No noise or bad odors
- Easy to breed

Disadvantages:
- Requires high humidity for best results, which makes it susceptible to mite infestation

King Mealworm Beetle/ Superworm (*Zophobas morio*)

This large beetle in Germany, (Fig. 47) ranges widely in South and Central America. Since about 1977 it has been known; it was introduced to Germany by Mr. Pepe Alcaraz, Köln. At first, it was only bred and shown in insect exhibits at zoos, then it found its way into the vivarium enthusiast community as a welcome new food animal. By now, it is firmly established, both with commercial breeders as well as with their customers. For example, we would like to mention Mr. Lehnert, from Heidenheim, who has for the first time raised Eurasian Hoopes without losses; thanks to superworms, as he assures us. We share his joy over his success!

Description: This dull-black beetle is 3-3.4 cm long and 1-1.2 cm wide. The head is somewhat longer than wide, the antennae are thin and 7-8 mm long. The scutellum is rectangular and only slightly rounded in the front. The 2 cm long elytra taper into a tip at the rear end and show lengthwise grooves. Males and females can be

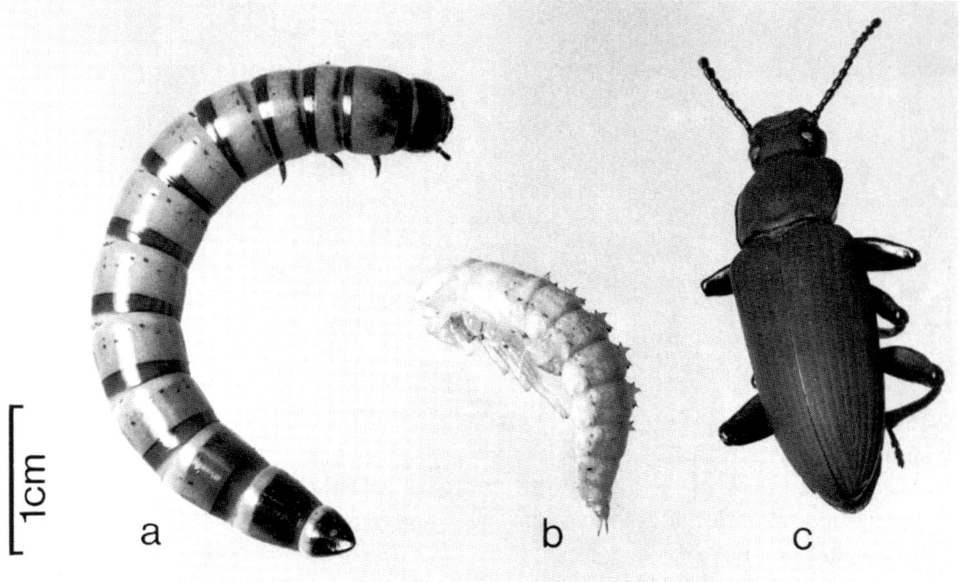

Fig. 47 King mealworm beetle (*Zophobas morio*). a) Larva before last molt, b) pupa, c) male.

114

distinguished by the shape of their heads; the male's head is 4.5-5 mm wide, the female's only 3.5-4 mm. If the beetles are touched, they secrete a milky-white foul-smelling liquid at their neck.

The glassy, white, slimy eggs of 1.2 to 1.4 mm length hatch 2-2.5 mm long, wheat-yellow larvae. They reach a length of 5.5-6 cm at a diameter of 5-7 mm and weigh in average 1.5 g. They are hearty chunks! The three rearmost segments and the head of the larger larvae are brown. All other segments have a brown band on their rear edge, and the middle segments also show small spots. The underside is wheat yellow, and the final segment is dark brown. If the larvae are grabbed tightly, they spray a clear, bitter-tasting liquid from their anus.

Development Times: At a preferred temperature of 27-29°C *Zophobas morio* requires 3½-4 months to develop. However, the size of the larvae compensates for this long development time. The eggs incubate for 8-12 days, and these voracious larvae reach their full size after 6-8 weeks. If they are kept separately, they will pupate 2-3 weeks later. The pupa rests for 2-3 weeks. The beetles start to mate 2 weeks after they emerge, and the females lay their first eggs a week later, 20-60 per clutch. Even at 18°C this beetle will still reproduce, but development takes about 1 year. If kept at their preferred temperature, the beetles live for about 1 year. In this time a female lays at least 1500 eggs.

Containers, Substrate, and Equipment: Breeding *Zophobas morio* requires containers that are impervious to moisture with smooth sides, like plastic or PVC tubs or aquariums. They should measure at least 35 x 20 x 20 cm. Wooden cages are out of the question, as the larvae will chew through them.

The beetles fly rarely, but adding a lid makes the breeding container escape-proof. At least half of the cover should be make of screen.

The substrate for the larvae must be lose and aerated, retain heat, and absorb and store moisture. All these requirements are met by a mixture of equal parts of unfertilized peat moss and sawdust. We were not as successful with other substrates, such as forest soil, garden soil, or finely chopped moss. The sawdust of leafy or coniferous trees should not be obtained from cabinet makers or carpenters, as it will almost always contain traces of finishes, glues, and solvents, which are deadly for the larvae as we learned the hard way. Even when getting the sawdust from sawmills care must be taken that it does not originate from trees that have been treated with insecticides. R. Wicker successfully uses a substrate made from ground up bark, into which the females also lay their eggs; and D. Schulten uses the coarsest Vermiculite, the grain size that is usually used as a packaging material (oral comm.).

If the king mealworms cannot be housed in a boiler room or a breeding cabinet, the desired temperature is best reached with a heating pad underneath the container. Like the rose weevil (*Pachnoda butana*) *Zophobas morio* likes to bask under an incandescent light bulb or an infrared heat emitter. Both must be installed outside the container. One to two infrared heat emitters can be sufficient as the only sources of heat.

The females attach their eggs in small clumps to a suitable medium; in the wild into cracks and small crevices where they are protected from predatory beetles. A cracked piece of wood, pieces of cork bark (Schulten, oral comm.), short pieces of rolled up corrugated cardboard (Stark, 1989), 3-4 pieces of cork tile, or a stack of tightly packed egg cartons will all work; the latter two should be placed vertically, and all should be placed directly onto the substreate. The egg laying substrates must be kept moist at all times so that the eggs will not dry out and die.

The containers are filled with about 7 cm of lightly moist substrate. Further setup decisions depend on whether at least 10 containers are started for large-scale breeding or only one container for small-scale breeding. For small-scale breeding, in addition to the egg-laying areas, some branches should be added for the beetles to walk on. To prevent the introduction of pests, the branches should be rinsed with boiling water or stored dry for a while.

For large-scale breeding, each container that contains beetles should be outfitted with a frame made of PVC or wood that is treated with Reposal. The underside of this frame is covered with a screen made of steel mesh or aluminum mesh (mesh size 0.8 mm). Mosquito screen is not fine enough and the beetles can stick their heads through and eat the eggs. The small larvae can also climb through and end up being eaten by the beetles.

This frame is placed on top of the 4 cm layer of egg cartons that covers the substrate completely. The females will lay their eggs through the screen in circles around the peaks of the egg cartons. On top of the frame another 2-3 egg cartons are stacked for the beetles.

Food: Like most other mealworm beetles, *Zophobas morio* eats both plant as well as animal matter. They can be fed with greens and fruit, such as lettuce, dandelion leaves, carrots, bananas, apples, pears, or oranges. In addition, a mixture of 300 g oats, 200 g soy meal, 30-40 g of brewers or dry yeast, and 50 g milk powder makes a good dry food. Small portions of this mixture are moistened with enough water that small balls can shaped. Mixtures made of other types of grains can also be used. The larvae will also eat wood mulch and dead roots; the beetles like animal matter as a supplement, such as moistened dry food for cats or dogs, dead night-crawlers, and snails. They especially like fresh fish, but it must be consumed within a few hours. All the food for the larvae and beetles, which should be replaced every 1-2 days, is offered in a kind of wire bowl. To make one, an hourglass-shaped bowl is made from a piece of nonrusting wire mesh of 5-6 mm mesh size. This is placed on the substrate filled with food. The animals can reach the food from all sides without scattering it all around the container where it would become a source of rot. This also makes it easier to determine the required amounts of food. Only the wood mulch is mixed into the substrate.

Breeding Conditions:
Light: The animals need little light and avoid sunlight, but they appreciate radiant heat. Even complete darkness probably does not affect reproduction.
Temperature: The best temperature for breeding is 27-29°C. The maximum temperature for larvae is 32°C, and 35-38°C for beetles. At 15-16°C reproduction ceases.
Humidity: The substrate should always be slightly moist; the larvae avoid dry substrate. A good hatch rate is reached at

60% air humidity, but the humidity can be as high as 90%. It is necessary to mist the container daily.

The water requirements of *Zophobas morio* are met by their food.

Notes:

Small-scale breeding: With a breeding stock of 40-60 beetles and as many larvae, animals can soon be harvested for feeding. However, even with 20 beetles and a little patience breeding can be successful. Once a breeding setup is established, 200-250 beetles can produce up to 800 g of larvae weekly; that is, 500-600 of them. This harvest is quite sizable, especially since it can be accomplished using just one container. Also this probably is the size limit for the hobbyist. A 50 x 30 x 30 cm container would be fully loaded and the substrate must be filled in to 10-12 cm to provide enough room for the larvae. This many larvae also produce profuse amounts of feces. Regular cleaning is necessary, about every 3 weeks if the containers are used to capacity. The substrate must be sifted with a sieve of mesh size 3-3.5 mm. Peat moss lumps, beetles, and the large larvae remain in the sieve. All of this is transferred into a second breeding container, or temporarily into a bucket until the container has been cleaned. The substrate is replenished and then everything is reassembled. In the discarded substrate, quite a few young larvae can be found. For this reason, it is either returned to the first cage or put into a smaller container (if only one breeding setup is purchased). After 3 weeks these larvae, which of course have to be fed, will be large enough that they will stay in a sieve of 1.5-2 mm mesh size. The remaining substrate is pretty much feces and sawdust.

If coarse Vermiculite is used as the substrate, a sieve of 5 mm mesh size is used through which all the larvae, big ones included, will fall (Schulten, oral comm.). If the population density in the container with the adult larvae is too high, they will not pupate, which means that larvae can be bred in large numbers ahead of time, then kept up to a year, however, with some losses (S. Rykena, oral comm.). However, this requires directed and separate growing of beetles for breeding stock. This is most likely to succeed if each larva is reared separately, for example in an empty yogurt cup or a similar small plastic cup. (They can chew through soft plastic containers). Yogurt cups can be stacked efficiently; 2 cm rim-height is enough for the larvae. It is important to allow them to pupate and develop in a dark, quiet place. This takes about 4-5 weeks at 25°C. The beetles are only moved into the breeding container after their exoskeleton is hard and black. Alternatively, egg cartons can be stacked into a transparent container and one larva placed into each cup. This container is placed into a quiet, dark, and warm corner, and the beetles can be removed when they start to walk around.

Large-scale breeding: Just like the yellow mealworm beetles, the beetles and the various stages of larvae must be separated. This makes for quite a bit of work.

For the beetles, the containers are fitted with frames and they are fed bran or coarsely milled grain and fresh foods. Every week the frame is moved to a new (freshly prepared) container and food is added. As soon as the larvae hatch, they receive the same foods as the beetles. Sifting, replenishing of the substrate, and feeding until the larvae are fully grown are the same as for the yellow mealworm beetle.

A climate-controlled breeding room is desirable and should be kept at a temperature of 27-30°C and an air humidity of 70-90%. For safety reasons, any lamps and all electrical wiring must be approved for use in humid environments.

Storage: Adult larvae can be kept without feeding for at most two months, preferably at room temperature; the minimum temperature is 15°C. The lavae must be mixed with at least the same amount in volume of dry bran.

Pests and Diseases: Since breeding requires a tropical climate, the occurrence of pests and diseases will come as no surprise. The substrate is an ideal breeding ground for mites and bacteria. In all cases the breeding containers should be closely watched.

Feeding: The larvae are so large that they can be found easily in the substrate and picked by hand. Alternatively, a small net can be used to sift a handful of substrate. Beetles and larvae cannot escape from smooth bowls, but any round bowls must be at least 1 cm taller than the larvae are long. Since they crawl around restlessly, they will soon attract the attention of the vivarium animals. Of course, they can also be offered using any of the other described methods, however, tweezers must be pinched strongly to prevent escape. Because of their size, the larvae of *Zophobas morio* are especially suitable for larger invertebrates (e.g., bird spiders), salamanders, lizards, birds, and small mammals. Careful! Escaped larvae can cause damage in terrariums and bird cages by eating eggs and baby birds.

Advantages and Disadvantages:
Advantages:
- Large, easily digestible larvae
- No smell, no noise
- Can be bred where people live
- Medium amount of work

Disadvantages:
- Long development times
- For large-scale operations a climate-controlled room is required

Bean Weevil (*Acanthoscelides obtectus*)

Most seed weevils lay their eggs on the green pods of legumes, or, as for example *A. obtectus*, into pods that have already turned yellow. The larvae drill either first through the pod or directly into the developing seed; they hatch from the ripe seeds. The bean weevils will also lay their eggs among ripe dry beans and the larvae develop inside. This is why they are a dreaded pest in storerooms and pantries. The United States is probably the country of origin (Zacher, 1955) of the bean weevil but by now it can be found worldwide. It is likely that *A. obtectus* traveled through Spain into the rest of Europe inside infested seeds. Even in the cooler regions of Northern Germany it has been found outdoors, occasionally since 1931, more often after WW II (Zacher, 1955; Zachariae, 1958). It still threatens dwarf beans and runner beans in all of central Europe. *A. obtectus* can survive at both high and low temperatures, and it reproduces in fields as well as in storage rooms. This is why it has spread worldwide.

If you should get your hands on any other kinds of seed weevils (from dried seeds),

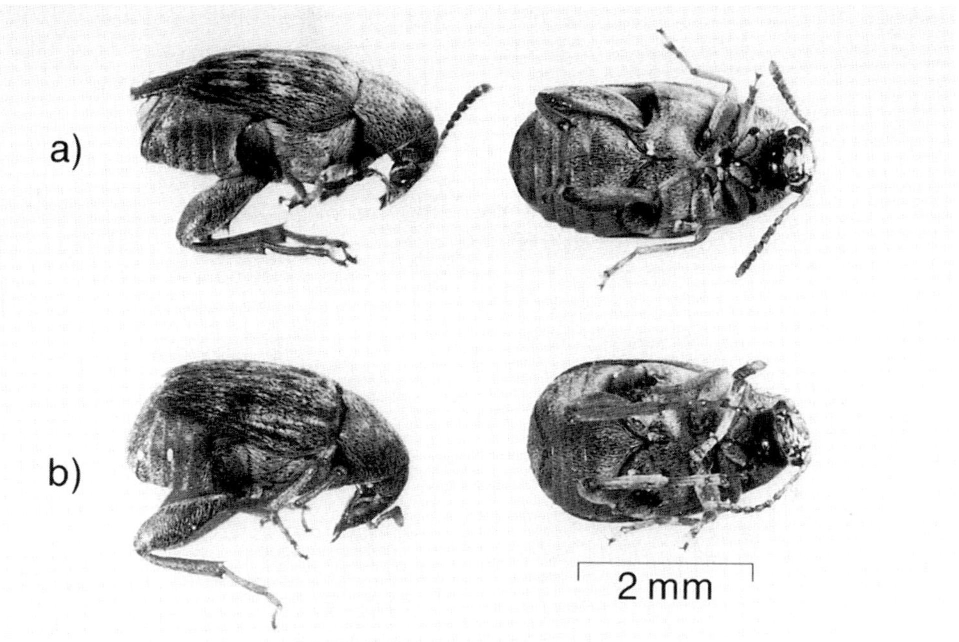

Fig. 48 Bean weevil (*Acanthoscelides obtectus*). a) Female b) male.

they can be bred in the same way as the bean weevil. Pohlman (1964) found not only *Acanthoscelides obtectus* in a bag of beans at a friend's house, but also what probably were Mexican bean weevils (*Zabrotes subfasciatus*). Fish and frogs love to eat both species—and probably others, too.

Description: The beetles are 3-4 mm long, about 1.4 mm high, and 2 mm wide, green-gray-brown colored and covered with hair; the smaller animals are usually males. The end of the male's abdomen is curved more than that of the female (Fig. 48). The elytra are shorter than the abdomen; they show thick black lengthwise stripes and a faint light and dark mottling. The scutellum has black spots. The antennae on the trunk-like,

elongated head are bout 1.5 mm long. The legs and the pygidium shine reddish. Details of coloring and morphologically distinctive features can only be seen at 10x magnification.

The club-like, 0.6-0.7 mm long eggs and the larvae are white. When they hatch, they measure 0.52-0.56 mm; they have 6 legs, and their pygidium forms an anal proleg. These tiny larvae can actually move about 20 cm (Zacher, 1930)! In order to drill into a seed, the larvae require something to push against. Therefore, they preferably drill into the seeds from below or from the sides of a container; they cannot get into loosely spaced beans (Zacher, 1930). After their first molt (of a total of four), the larvae become legless. To finish their development, they make a tunnel out to just inside of skin of the seed, which can be seen as a small, dark spot, a "window." This is where the beetle will emerge by cutting through the skin and pushing to the outside after escaping from its light-brown pupa.

Development Times: At about 20°C a new generation of beetles develops in 11 to 12 weeks. About a week after they emerge from their pupae, the beetles become lively, crawl and fly around, mate, and live in between the beans and lay their eggs, loosely and one at a time. After about 10 weeks "windowed" beans can be spotted. The beetles live for about 3-4 weeks. These measurements agree with Menusan (1934) who at 21°C notes 10 days for embryo development, 46 days for larval development and pupation, and a 19-day lifespan for the beetles. At 27°C his experiments yielded 6 + 28 + 10 days (all times rounded) respectively, which we have confirmed 50 years later. At the high temperature of 27-30°C, the short lifespan of the adult beetles is noteworthy. Since they are the only stage harvested for food, they must be harvested at the right time; that is, about one week after they emerge from the beans. By then, the females have already laid quite a few eggs. The total number of eggs is around 40-60, which is also noted in the literature (Zacher, 1930; Zachariae, 1958). Under ideal conditions, a female can deposit about 75 eggs (Menusan, 1934).

Containers, Substrate, and Development: Fill several jars of ½-2 l with 3-4 cm of beans; add the beetle breeding stock, and close the jars with a fitted lid or plastic wrap that is held in place with a rubber band. The lid should have small (1 mm max.) holes or a wire-mesh window (0.6 mm mesh size) that is glued or soldered to the lid. Doubly layered nylon is only a temporary solution, as the beetles will eat holes into it within a few days and escape.

Food: The larvae eat practically nothing but the beans, only their seminal leaves, but not the seedlings, whether they are hiding in a white, green, black, red, or spotted bean (Fig. 49). Even in chickpeas they develop 100% (Herford, 1936). In other legumes, such as peas, lentils, and soybeans, the rate of success is moderate to none.

The beans should have a water content of 10-12%; store-bought beans are usually drier. The desired water content can be achieved by wetting 850 g of beans with 150 ml of water, after the seeds have first been dried at 40-50°C until their weight does not change anymore (Wyninger, 1974). For practical purposes, 850 g of bean seeds can be rinsed with 100-120 ml of water until they are evenly wet. When the outside has dried again, they can be added to the breeding jar.

Under the conditions that the bean weevils find in stored beans, they do not eat at all. This explains their short lifespan. Zachariae (1958) observed bean weevils outdoors, how they licked nectar from flowers that allowed them access, and how they cut the green pods of bean plants to lick the seeping juice. Thus nourished they lived through the summer, until the females laid their eggs into the ripening, yellowing bean pods. These observations suggest the conclusion that feeding honey-water will keep the beetles alive longer. We did not investigate this but observed that they like to drink the honey-water.

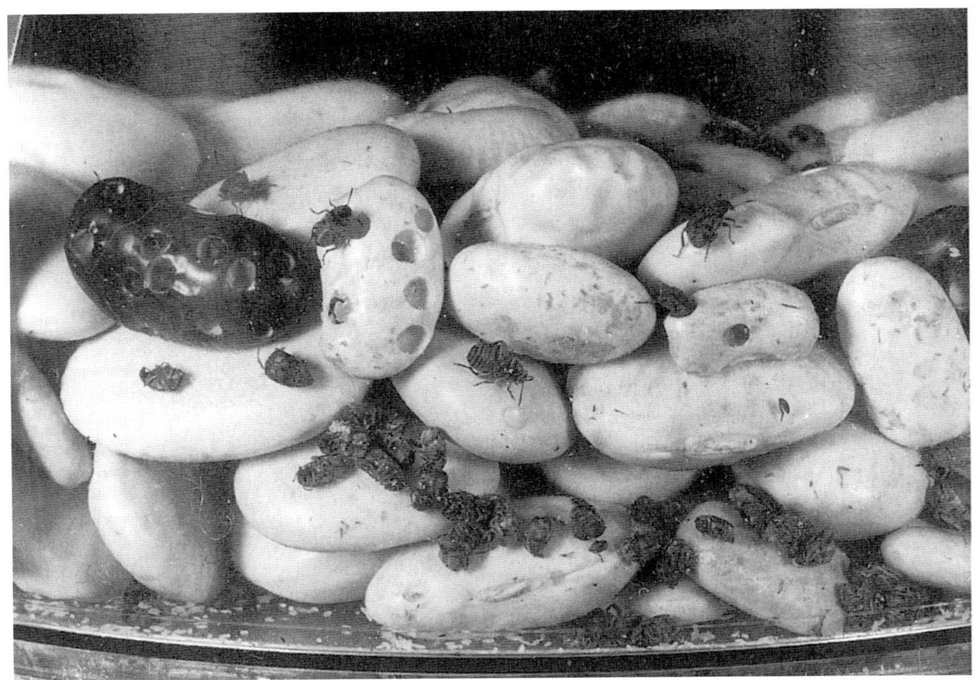

Fig. 49 View into breeding jar for bean weevils.

Breeding Conditions:

Light: The breeding jars can be placed in the dark or light. If they stand in a very bright spot, the beetles are especially lively and fly towards the light source.

Temperature: At a range of 20-28°C the beetles reproduce well and rather fast; at a temperature of almost 25°C most of the beetles will hatch (Menusan, 1936). They can reproduce when temperatures are 17–31°C (Menusan, 1934).

Humidity: Even though several experiments determined that the optimal air humidity is 80-90% (e.g., Menusan, 1934, 1936; Horber, 1950), the chances of mold increase with each percentage point, so that a suboptimal level of 50-70% humidity appears to be the best solution. Under no circumstances should condensation droplets form on the beans. If the larvae grow at a higher humidity level, the beetles will be larger than those that have developed under drier conditions (Menusan, 1936). The humidity should not fall below 25%.

Notes: After the breeding containers have been set up, one only has to wait until the next generation hatches. Up to 15 larvae can develop in the smaller beans, in larger beans up tot 30. Once the beans have multiple holes, new beans should be added and the setup may be divided up into two jars. Dead beetles, feces, and shell pieces accumulate over time. About 3 weeks after no more living beetles are in a jar, its contents are poured into a sieve, shaken until the beans are clean of debris, and placed into a new glass. Less work cannot be expected from any breeding setup! A living breeding setup smells fruity-sweet, one that has gone bad will smell stale-sweet.

Pests and Diseases: The setup must not become moldy since the beetles and larvae will die. We know of one parasitic mite, *Pediculoides ventricosus*. Affected beetles will die, so that an infested setup will spoil. If this mite is discovered, we recommend destruction of the breeding setup. This mite can also be passed on to people and cause skin diseases (Zacher, 1930).

Feeding: Unlike with the other beetles we discussed, here the adult beetles are the food item. The larvae could only be harvested by gently opening the beans. Food beetles are tossed into the water or tightly locked terrariums since they can fly and climb smooth walls and cannot be restrained in a bowl. As Pohlmann (1964) mentions, small frogs and fish that eat flying food, as well as small lizards, like these beetles for variety.

It is difficult to catch single beetles from the jar since they let themselves drop when touched and scurry deeper and deeper into the beans. It is easiest to scoop beans and beetles into a separate container and place it in the terrarium. If the beetles are needed separately, for example, for fish, they can be sifted out.

Advantages and Disadvantages:

Advantages:

- Very small amount of work

Disadvantages:

- Pest on legumes; keep breeding setups away from the pantry, at the least in a different room
- Beetles are difficult to catch

Rose Weevil
(*Pachnoda butana*)

Description: The strong body of the West African rose weevil (Fig. 50) appears angular and egg-shaped. It is about 22-25 mm long, 13-15 mm wide, and 9 mm thick. The beetle shows pretty markings in strong warm yellow and silky brown-red colors. A yellow rim surrounds the scutellum. Scutellum and elytra are brownred to half their length, with a yellow seam on the side; the rear half displays a washed out red brown spot. The underside of the body is shiny black. Males and females can be distinguished by their antennae: the male has seven leaf-like lamella, the female only five.

The white, spherical eggs of 1.5-1.8 mm diameter turn light brown shortly before they hatch. The larvae hatch with a length of 3 mm and can grow to 50 mm in length and 10 mm in diameter. They look like June bug larvae; they are colored dirty white except for the red brown head with its strong mouthparts. The larvae have

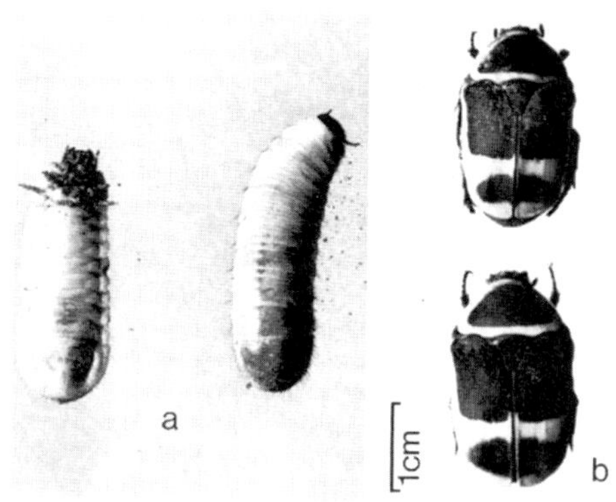

Fig. 50 Rose weevil (*Pachnoda butana*). a) Larvae, b) beetles.

some light-brown hairs and show a noticeable skin bulges on their flanks. Their way of moving on smooth surfaces is rather peculiar: the larva rolls up, turns on its back, and crawls off.

Development Times: The complete development time is 10-11 weeks, an extremely short time span for a rose weevil. However, temperatures of 28-30°C are required. The larvae hatch after 10-14 days, reach their full size after 35-45 days, and pupate for 2 days. They rest in their pupae for up to 10 days, and the beetle remains in the cocoon for 3 days until its exoskeleton has hardened. After 4-6 days the beetles reach sexual maturity, and 7 days later the females begin laying their eggs. They can deposit up to 70 eggs, 8-12 per clutch. The males live 6-8 weeks, the females up to 5 months.

Even at 18°C these beetles will still reproduce, but the development time extends over three quarters of a year. The beetles also live longer.

Containers, Substrate, Equipment: The larvae of the rose weevil live in the ground, and the beetles fly well. They require breeding containers that are at least 40-50 cm tall with a lid; best are large plastic or glass terrariums. A container of 40 x 30 x 40 cm has room for about 200 larvae and 60-80 beetles.

The container receives heat and light from an incandescent light bulb that is mounted on the outside and above—the beetles like to bask under it—and from a heating pad that is placed underneath to heat the substrate to the desired temperature.

The substrate consists of a mixture of equal parts of forest soil, unfertilized peat moss, leaves, clay, and sand. To make sure no pests or uninvited guests are introduced, the substrate should be steamed. To do this it is moistened, spread onto a baking sheet, and baked for 15 minutes at 130°C. The substrate is then filled to a height of 25 cm into the container. Some branches or a root is added for climbing; these, too, are preferably rinsed with boiling water first to prevent the introduction of pests.

Food: Rose weevils eat primarily plant materials, especially flowers of all kinds, as well as rose and blackberry leaves. In captivity, they can be fed on sweet fruit like bananas, pears, oranges, peaches, and grapes. The fruit is cut open and placed on top of the substrate in a shallow bowl. Orange slices can also be skewered onto branches. Even better development and growth result if they are fed prepared waxworm food.

The larvae eat primarily the wood of dead leaf trees, for example, of oak, beech, linden, chestnut, or willow trees. The wood is buried into the dirt, as well as pieces of fruit and carrot, which are also eaten. We have observed that adding clay or clay-containing dirt promotes growth of the larvae.

Breeding Conditions:
Light: The beetles require a day-night rhythm. Moderate light during the day suffices since they are mostly nocturnal. An incandescent light bulb is the best source of light; it also warms the con-tainer. A 40-watt bulb is usually sufficient.
Temperature: As mentioned earlier, for a high-yield setup the temperature must be 28-30°C. The substrate temperature should not be higher than 30°C since the larvae cannot tolerate higher temperatures. A 25-watt heating pad probably suffices for the recommended cages. At temperatures below 18°C, reproduction ceases.

Humidity: The soil mixture must be moist at all times, but without standing water. If the dirt dries out too much, the eggs will not hatch. The beetles are misted every 2-3 days. On the substrate, air humidity should be 80-90%.

Notes: *Pachnoda butana* has only been bred since 1975, primarily for exposition in insect zoos. Few people breed them as food animals, most of them probably because this beetle is so pretty.

After setting up the breeding containers with heat and food, 30 beetles, preferably 10 males and 20 females, are added as breeding stock. If food larvae are not needed as soon as possible, breeding can also be initiated with only 5-10 animals; the relatively high price of these beetles might influence this choice. Soon after it may be possible to observe them mating in the dark.

The females disappear a few days later into the ground to deposit their eggs. The eggs are deposited at the bottom of the container and covered with a protective layer of dirt so that they are difficult to find; it is better not to dig in the substrate.

For the next 7 weeks feedings are only needed every 1-2 days; leftovers and the top-most layer of soil with the feces are removed, and the temperature and humidity are checked and regulated. When they pupate, the larvae construct a cocoon by mixing dirt and sand particles with their saliva; it is usually attached to the bottom or the sides of the breeding container. Once the first generation of beetles hatches, the question is whether to increase the breeding stock. If so, a second terrarium is equipped and half the beetles are moved there. Otherwise, a portion of the now growing larvae can be used for food.

In a container of 50 x 35 x 50 cm 80-120 beetles that will reproduce fast enough to leave 50-100 larvae per week for harvesting can be kept. This is a relatively small amount, but a monitor lizard of 50 cm length will be quite full after eating 10 large larvae.

If the container is stocked with about 100 beetles, the top 10 cm of the substrate must be removed and replaced weekly. Before the old substrate is discarded, it should be sifted for larvae.

About every 6 months a complete cleaning is necessary. The easiest way to do this is to set up a second breeding container. Then the beetles that have not dug into the substrate are moved first. Be careful: when they start to pump their abdomens, they are about to take off. Then the substrate is removed, layer by layer, and the beetles and larvae are picked out by hand. The larvae move down and collect at the bottom. The cocoons are gently pried off with a razor blade and moved to the new container. The lowest layer of dirt, about 15 cm, is reused, so that the eggs and smallest larvae are not wasted.

If only one breeding container is available, all the animals are temporarily stored in a bucket while the container is emptied, cleaned, and set up again for their return.

Pests and Diseases: For the time that rose weevils have been bred, no diseases have shown up. We have not noticed any deaths of larvae or beetles for unknown reasons. Like any insect breeding setup, it can become infested by mites. Cleanliness and regular renewal of the substrate are the best prevention.

Feeding: The larvae are best offered from a round, smooth bowl with a 2-3 cm rim from which they cannot escape. They can also be offered with tweezers or—for tame animals—by hand. The larvae should not be allowed to dig into the terrarium substrate.

Up until now we have only used the larvae as food—the beetles are just too beautiful! Larger lizards, toads, and frogs welcome rose weevil larvae as an enrichment of their diet. Many small mammals, for example bush babies and slow loris will accept this treat with enthusiasm.

Otherwise, little experience exists and many other vivarium animals might love rose weevils if given the opportunity to taste them.

Advantages and Disadvantages:

Advantages:

- Moderate amount of work
- Large, fat larvae make good supple-mental food
- No risk breeding in apartments and houses

Disadvantages:

- Requires relatively large amount of space
- Not an all-round food animal because of slow reproduction

Flies (Diptera)

The translation of the Latin name of the order Diptera means "two-wingers," which points to a property they all share. Only the frontal pair of wings is formed, the rear pair appears only as a pair of buds. The about 90,000 species of flies are small to very small insects whose general appearance is well known. There are the mosquitoes, which can transmit dangerous diseases, and species like the housefly, fruit fly, and blowfly that can often be found indoors. Suitable food

flies are known from four families: the Drosophilidae with the genus *Drosophila*, the Muscidae with *Fannia* and *Musca*, the Calliphoridae with *Calliphora* and *Lucilia*, as well as the Sarcophagidae with *Sarcophaga*. These flies all have mouthparts adapted for licking and sucking. They can dissolve solid particles with their saliva and eat them just like liquids. The adults and the maggots, legless larvae, eat both plant as well as animal foods.

Small Fruit Fly (*Drosophila melanogaster*) Large Fruit Fly (*Drosophila funebris*) Large Wingless Fruit Fly (*Drosophila hydei*)

Description: *Drosophila melanogaster* reaches a length of 2-2.5 mm and 1 mm in diameter, and is colored light brown with a shiny yellow or red-brown abdomen. The rear rim of each segment is dark brown; in the male the last two segments are black, in the female black brown. The eyes shine red. The two colorless, 2 mm long wings are iridescent depending on the light, especially in males looking to mate.

Out of 0.5 mm long and 0.2 mm wide eggs with two string-like attachments hatch larvae of the same size, which grow, through 3 molts, to 5 mm length and 1 mm diameter. The mature maggots settle down somewhere outside the cultivation medium, shrink, and pupate into 3 mm long pupae, which, as they age change, color from light brown to a prominent red brown.

Thanks to the fast succession of generations, the high mutation rate, and hereditary mutations, the fruit fly is a favorite research animal for geneticists. As a food animal, the vestigial form is of significance. *Drosophila funebris* grows larger, to 3-3.5 mm, with wings of the same length. The head and thorax are medium to dark brown, the eyes dark wine red, the abdomen appears light brown yellow on the underside and dark brown on top—in the male almost dark brown with lighter narrow banding on the back and the front rim of each segment. A light stripe along the center of the body reaches across the abdomen. The female can be easily recognized by its bloated abdomen after she is a few days old.

The 0.6-mm-long oval eggs have four threadlike attachment organs. The up to 6 mm long and 1 mm thick maggots pupate into 4 mm long and 1 mm thick reddish brown pupae.

The most prominent feature of *Drosophila hydei* are their large red shining eyes. The size and colors of the flies, eggs, maggots, and pupae are the same as for *Drosophila funebris*. Most of the maggots pupate at or on the surface of the substrate.

This species is of interest to the vivarium enthusiast because a form that has wings but cannot fly is available. It is sometimes offered under the name Afghan fruit fly.

Development Times: At a room temperature of 20-22°C the small and large fruit flies develop at about the same rate. The females mate within 24 hours after emerging from their pupae, no later. From the third day they lay eggs, about 300-350 within 16 days, if fed well. After 1-2 days the minuscule maggots hatch, which pupate after 5-7 days and rest for 4-6 days, so that the next generation of flies hatches after about 15 days. The lifespan of the flies is 8-10 weeks; they lay eggs for about 4 weeks.

At the same temperature, the cycle for *D. hydei* is about twice as long; that is, 34-40 days. The hatched flies only start laying after 11-13 days, the maggots hatch 2 days later and need 11-13 days to grow up. After 10-12 days the adult flies will emerge. This form is as fertile as the others; one female lays about 22 eggs per day, for about 6 weeks, during the 3rd to 8th weeks of life. Thereafter egg production is reduced. Life expectancy is about 10 weeks at 20-22°C.

Containers, Substrate, and Equipment: Smaller glass or plastic jars of about 8-12 cm diameter and 12-20 cm height are best for breeding fruit flies, as for example jam, honey, or pickle jars. Cans do not work as well because they make checking on the maggots harder. Large jars of over 2 l volume ha are too unwieldy. Plastic laboratory jars that are bout 10 cm high and 5 cm in diameter with a foam plug are recommended. Stein (1964) recommends rectangular plastic containers into which a small pipe is fitted on the side, in the upper third of the box. A hole is cut into the lid and covered with fabric.

The cultivation medium is the substrate; about 1-2 cm is filled into the container. Wood-wool, pieces of egg carton or paper strips are loosely added on top, which serve as resting places and hiding places for the pupae. Alternatively, a plastic grille can be used (Schöpfel, 1978).

The jar is always sealed with a 20 cm long piece of nylon stockingthat is pulled over the glass and fastened with two (!) rubber bands that are twisted around into other multiple times (Fig. 51). It is best to use the

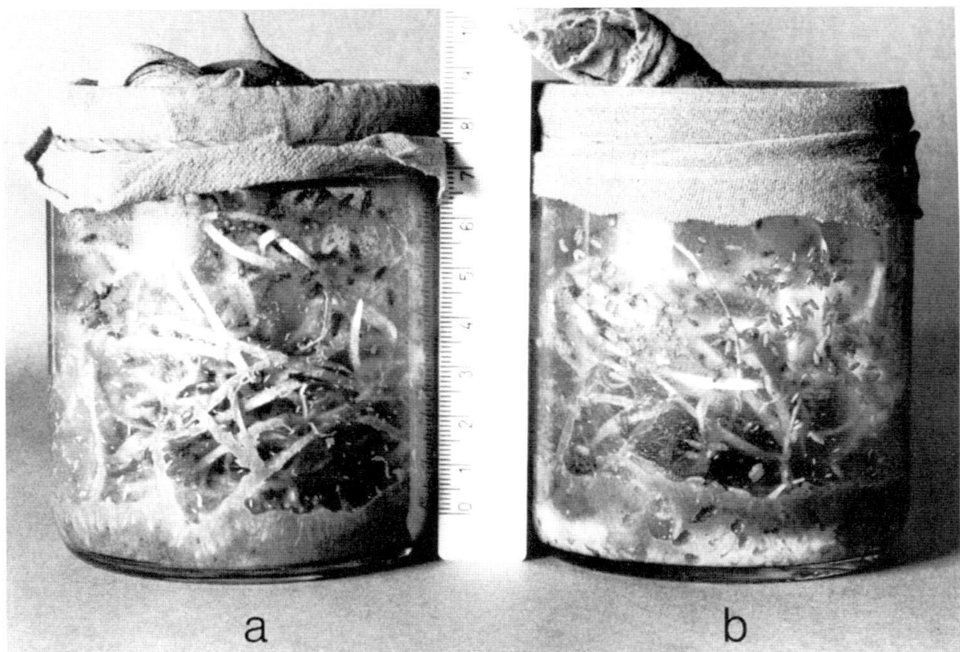

Fig. 51 *Drosophila* breeding jars. a) Large fruit fly (*Drosophila funebris*), b) small fruit fly (*Drosophila melanogaster*).

ankle section of the nylon stocking since its narrower opening fits tightly over the jar. For fruit flies that are incapable of flight the jar can be closed with cotton wool, a foam stopper, a piece of fabric, or a lid with air holes or a gauze-covered opening, especially for smaller jars with few animals. **Food**: As long as fruit flies are being bred, there will always be new recipes for the food paste. The most diverse mixtures yield good results if one knows what fruit flies eat. Fruit flies eat primarily yeasts, some bacteria—for example, vinegar bacteria—molds, and the fermentation products from overripe fruit. The best reproductive rate is reached in a mildly acidic substrate. Therefore, the paste needs to be made from (1) fruit or sugar, (2) wine or fruit vinegar, (3) yeast or brewer's yeast and (4) binders, so that it is not too liquid. The maggots have to breathe and can only use the top layer of the substrate if it is too liquid.

1. If sugar is not used by itself, mashed banana is a staple food that is available all year at a good price. Also suitable are apples, applesauce, carrots, potatoes, grated pears, all kinds of plums and grapes (cut and mashed). The fruit must be fully ripe, can be overripe (e.g., kiwis), but must not be rotten or moldy.

2. Both types of vinegar are equally suitable.

3. Brewer's yeast—available at health food stores—has the advantage that it keeps much longer and the paste does

127

not ferment as much.

4. As binders bread crumbs, semolina, cotton wool, peat moss (Körber, 1984), ground up grains, oats, or bran can be used. The last two are most susceptible to mold. Nipagin, which is available at drugstores, prevents molding. However, it has not been determined whether fruit flies that contain Nipagin will adversely affect the development of young frogs and lizards. If the breeding setups are carefully supervised, no Nipagin is necessary. It is advantageous to add some liquid vitamins or mineral powder to the mixture. Adding milk powder or prepared milk pudding makes old paste smell very bad.

The paste mixture should be semisolid. What does this mean? If the mixture stands for about one hour, no liquid should separate out. Over time, experience will help you recognize the right consistency. If the mixture gets too dry after a few days, it can be remoistened with some vinegar-water.

In some recipes it is stated that all ingredients except for the yeast and vitamins must be boiled. This effort is however unnecessary and has no advantages. Our setups should require as little time as possible! Here are two recipes. We especially recommend the first one without reservations; it approaches to the natural diet and we have used it for many years. It also produces a high yield: in 120 ml of the food mixture 65 ml of *D. hydei* can be cultivated.

Recipe for our cultivation medium:
  ½ banana
  ½ apple
  1 small carrot
  1 teaspoon brewer's yeast
  ½-1 tablespoon vinegar
  1 tablespoons bread crumbs or coarsely ground grains
  1 pinch of vitamin powder with calcium and trace elements (for 2 jars)

Cultivation medium according to Nestler (1960):
  1 small raw potato
  1 small apple or same amount of fruit leftovers
  1 teaspoon sugar
  1 teaspoon lanolin
  3 g baking yeast
  1 tablespoon oats
  1 small pinch of salt
  50-100 cm^3 milk

A new Drosophila instant food is now commercially available. It contains cellulose, apple flour, soy flour, minerals, trace elements, vitamins, amino acids, Nipagin, paprika flour, and beta-carotene. The composition is chosen such that not only the flies develop well, but the frogs and lizards that are fed with them will also absorb the additives for their own benefit. The instant powder is mixed with an equal volume of water, left to sit for 10 minutes, stirred, and filled into 3-4 cm high into jars.

Another food mixture for fruit flies consists of a base of Agar-Agar, a substance that is extracted from red algae and that swells when mixed with hot liquid and then solidifies, like gelatin. (Agar-Agar is available in health food and drug stores.) Lilge and van Meeuwen (1979) suggest the following preparation:
  10 g of Agar-Agar dissolved in 700 ml of hot water
  60 g of cane sugar, 120 g cornstarch, and 10 g yeast dissolved in 160 ml of cold water.

Both solutions are briefly boiled, then filled still warm and liquid to 1 cm into the jars.

It is advantageous that this substrate remains bonded to the glass once it cools, and it can be prepared in advance; the jars can be covered with aluminum foil and stored in the freezer. The smell during preparation is unpleasant.

Cultivation medium according to Stettler (1979):

> 300 ml water is cooked with 2 g Agar--Agar, 20 g sugar.
>
> 40 g of corn meal are added, brought to a boil, and filled into a pickling jar of 0.5 l volume.

Then 10 g of baking yeast are dissolved and poured on top of the substrate. Half a lemon or another fruit can be added. Additional recipes are mentioned by Mußler (1982), Vergossen (1985), Kofahl (1987), Suttner (1990), and Stute (1991) in the context of extensive breeding instructions and descriptions of their experiences.

Breeding Conditions:

Light: Some natural or artificial lighting is necessary.

Heat: Good results are seen at 20-23°C. This is an ideal temperature for *D. hydei*, which ceases to lay eggs at temperatures above 25°C (Siepe, oral comm.). For the other species, development time is shortest when they are kept at a temperature of 24-26°C.

Humidity: The cultivation medium must not dry out; this self-regulates for a favorable climate. If water condenses on the sides, the *D. hydei* get stuck easily and cannot free themselves. According to Wyniger (1974), 80-90% humidity is ideal.

Notes:

Small-scale breeding: Three to four jars are required for even the smallest amount of Drosophila needed to guarantee a steady supply. A bright spot with room temperature should be easy to find for them. The two large fruit flies can only be bred continuously and with a high yield in jars larger than ½ l (0.13 g); in the lab jars it is very difficult to keep the setup balanced. The first breeding jar is set up completely before the flies are added, about 50 for a laboratory jar and 300 for a 750 ml jar. After a week they will have laid so many eggs that they must be transferred to a new jar. If they stay in the first jar too long, the newest maggots will not be able to find enough food and will die, unless more food is added. In the second jar the flies remain again for 8 days, until they are harvested and used as food, or they are transferred to a third jar to increase the breeding stock. In the first jar the next generation of flies has hatched in the meantime, and they have run out of food. Therefore they are transferred into a prepared jar where they are allowed to fill their bellies and then they can be harvested (many more animals hatch than are required for continuation of the breeding cycle). After three weeks the first jar is cleaned out—the breeding setups are now established and running. For *D. hydei* the cycle is twice as long.

Maybe it appears nitpicky to insist on such a regular and precise schedule, but it is the best method for obtaining fruit flies regularly and in excellent condition. Especially for *D. hydei* with its long development time, it is recommended to overstock the jars at first with flies. This many flies will eat from the whole surface of the cultivation medium, which prevents the formation of mold, which grows primarily in spots that are undisturbed.

Once all these flies have reproduced so well that not all the maggots can find enough food in the remaining paste—a sign of this is when the maggots start to climb the sides of the glass—the cultivation medium plus maggots is distributed into several jars (after the flies have been removed) and food paste is added.

This species is very sensitive to underfeeding. If too many maggots eat depleted cultivation medium it can happen that all the flies will die within a day, unless they are moved to a new jar in time.

Many people shy away from breeding fruit flies that are capable of flight since they are afraid they will soon find fruit flies all over the house. However, an open bowl with food will attract all those flies; they cannot resist it, and with a bit of patience they can be controlled easily. With a little care and practice the flies can be transferred without losing any.

If the jar is covered with a nylon stocking, the stocking is unwound except for 1-2 turns. A second jar is placed next to it, and the open end of the nylon stocking fitted over it. The second jar is now held low in one hand and the first jar above it in the other hand, and the nylon-stocking tunnel is completely opened. The flies, attracted by bright light and encouraged by a few shakes, fly up and collect in the second jar. The first jar is put down, and the stocking pinched to keep flies from returning. The second jar is shaken so that the flies get confused; the nylon stocking can be pulled off and the jar quickly covered with the hand. The stocking is twisted to close the first jar. If the new jar is also for breeding, a nylon stocking is pulled over the hand and the jar, the jar shaken again, and then the hand removed (Fig. 52). It is important that the nylon stocking fits tightly around the jars and is long enough that it does not pull off during the whole process.

According to Stein (1964), the jar is placed in a box made of black cardboard with only one hole where the plug of the jar fits through. A small tube is fitted over the hole into which the flies will crawl looking for light. This method can also be used to easily move the flies into a new jar.

If the jars are closed off with pieces of fabric, as it used to be recommended, or with a plug of cotton wool, it is much harder to take it off and make contact with another jar whose opening must fit precisely. It is best to cool the flies down in the refrigerator first or to shake them hard (but then you will have to work very fast). Once enough flies are in the upper jar, two pieces of cardboard are inserted between the two openings, and the glasses can be separated, each covered with a piece of cardboard.

For those fruit flies that cannot fly, however, a plug is convenient to close the jars. The animals are simply shaken and poured into the new breeding jar, or into a jar with calcium powder and then into the terrarium or aquarium. Consider that holding the jar upside down, makes it more likely that the cultivation medium will fall out. However, it can be supported with a fork to keep it from falling out. Only jars with Agar-Agar medium can be turned upside down and shaken without worry. For larger jars with many flies, using the nylon-stocking method is best since it allows you to reach into the jar.

If several species of fruit flies are kept, care must be taken to keep them separate. Those that develop faster will otherwise outbreed the slower ones.

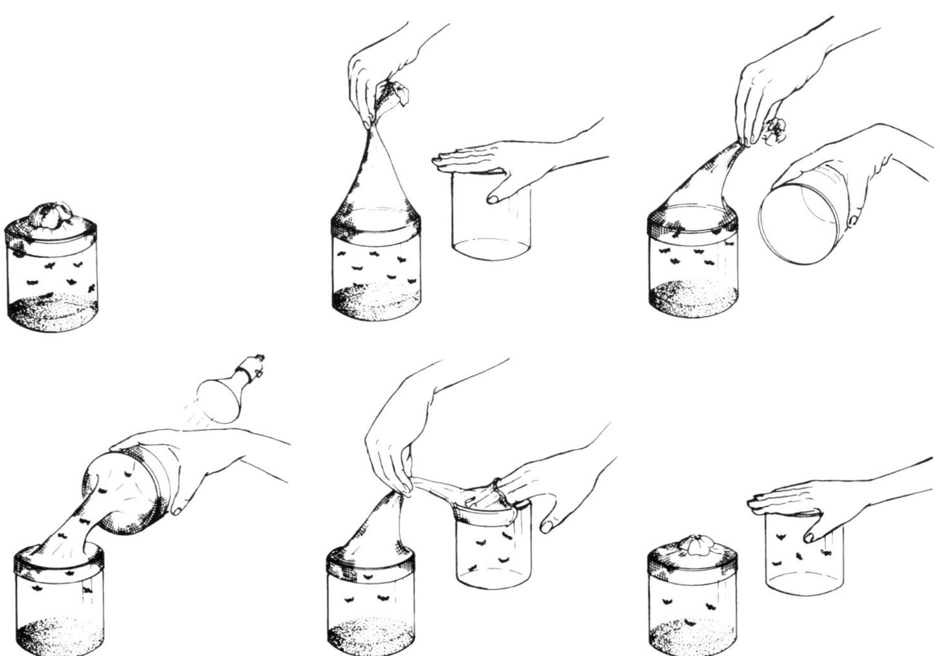

'Fig. 52 Transferring fruit flies.

Large-scale breeding: A large-scale breeding setup works very similarly to a small one. Of course, a much larger number of jars are used. Since it can become tedious to open and close the nylon covers for 10, 20, or more jars, several jars are placed into a larger container, for example, an aquarium, with a lid and a service door on the side. The door faces away from the light source or, even better, is covered with a gauze-tunnel. The gauze is glued to the frame so that the flies cannot collect between the rim and the fabric and be squashed when the fabric is tightened. To remove flies, there are two options. You can reach into the container, fit a lid or a plugged funnel over one of the jars, and carefully remove it. The flies are directly released into the terrarium or into a small jar where they are shaken with water or calcium powder depending on the intended use. Then the jar is placed back into the aquarium. Alternatively, the lid of the aquarium is fitted with a sliding door. A jar is fitted over the opening upside down, the sliding door is opened, and if a light shines from above, the flies will move up into the jar.

Stettler (1979) has instructions for a large breeding cage according to Nigg.

Pests and Diseases: The ever-present mites and the vinegar eels, which will munch on the cultivation medium, are worth mentioning. Clean breeding jars and regular and timely transfers into new jars keep them under control and might even get rid of them.

Mold can endanger breeding setups if a

carpet of mold spreads on the surface of the substrate before enough maggots have eaten their way into it.

Feeding: Only flies with full bellies are used as food. *D. melanogaster* and *D. funebris* require about 3-4 days, *D. hydei* about 5-8 days of feeding.

To feed fish, especially those living close to the surface, Drosophilae are unfortunately not used often enough even though they have been recommended for years. Here the wingless fruit fly is ideal. Winged animals are shaken with some water so that their wings get wet and they cannot fly. They are dropped into the fishtank in small amounts, in a corner where they cannot climb out onto plants right away. To be completely safe, they can be frozen first, but that removes their attraction as live food.

Small frogs and lizards are offered either the small or the large fruit flies. The terrarium should be constructed so that the flies cannot escape. The advantage of using the wingless form of *D. hydei* is that they are easy to handle.

It is often recommended to place a Drosophila jar into the terrarium and allow the inhabitants to serve themselves. This can be rather practical if it is not done all the time. Freshly metamorphosed amphibians and young lizards can easily get metabolic bone disease from lack of calcium if this is their primary food. It is therefore worth the trouble to feed small amounts at a time and dust them with calcium powder first.

To feed the maggots to vivarium animals, a bowl with a densely populated cultivation medium is placed into the cage. The vivarium animals will eat the maggots that crawl on the surface. Janssen (1986) has a suggestion for keeping small salamanders from getting stuck on the paste, or possibly sinking into it and drowning: A small glass or plastic tube of 5 cm diameter is filled almost to the rim with paste full of maggots that has been enriched with vitamins. The tube is closed with a nylon stocking and some rubber bands and placed into the terrarium, always in the same spot. When they search for a place to pupate, the maggots will crawl through the fabric and can easily be picked off by the salamanders that will soon recognize their source of easy food.

For fish, the larvae must be separated from the substrate; they are driven out of it by using heat. Depending on the needed amounts, the breeding jar, from which the flies have been removed, is placed on a lightly heated stove top (according to Fritz, 1967; if a finger can be placed onto the heater for 1 s without burning the stove is of the right temperature) or a small amount of the cultivation medium is removed and maggots are carefully removed with a brush, spatula, or small spoon and as they collect on the top and on the sides after about five minutes.

Fruit flies are essential for raising newly metamorphosed frogs, small diurnal lizards, as well as *Anolis*, day geckos, and chameleons. Surface-feeding fish like butterfly fish, hatched fish, and many egg-laying cichlids, as well as young spiders, and praying mantises among the invertebrates like them. Hummingbirds and other nectar-eating birds require fruit flies as part of a healthy diet; Chinese nightingales and a variety of finches also love them.

Advantages and Disadvantages:

Advantages:

- *Drosophila* can be bred in large

quantities at room temperature
- Little odor if they are transferred to new breeding jars frequently
- Require little space and only weekly care

Disadvantages:
- Escaped animals can be bothersome

Housefly
(Musca domestica)
Little Housefly
(Fannia canicularis)
Blowfly
(Calliphora erythrocephala)
Green Bottle Fly
(Lucilia caesar)
Flesh Fly
(Sarcophaga spec.)

Description: The gender of all flies can be determined by looking at the forehead, in addition to inspecting the abdomen, which is bigger and usually lighter colored in females: The eyes of the males are closer together and the forehead is therefore narrower than that of the females.

The maggots of all discussed species of flies, except those of *Fannia*, are cylindrical, whitish larvae whose body tapers towards the front end. An actual head cannot be recognized. The mouthparts are rather unusual and consist of several hooks that cannot be used for chewing. The maggots secrete saliva that breaks down proteins, which breaks the food down into a liquid form that they can slurp.

Musca domestica (Fig. 53): The housefly reaches a size of 6-8 mm and is gray with four dark, lengthwise stripes on the upper side of the thorax and yellow brown spots on the front part of the upper side of the abdomen.

The underside of the abdomen of the male is light gray, that of the female yellowish. Dark spots run along the sides and the middle of the abdomen. The end of each foot has an adhesive disk that is covered with many fine hairs. They are always moist so that the flies can hold on to completely smooth surfaces, even when upside down. Almost the whole body of the housefly is covered with hairs.

The cylindrical, milky white eggs are about 1 mm long, and so are the white, cylindrical maggots that hatch from them. They grow to a length of 9-11 mm. The barrel-shaped pupa which is 6.3 mm long and 2.5 mm thick in average changes color over time from light brown to medium brown to dark red brown.

A few years ago, at the University of Pavia (near Milan), Dr. Dieter Bretz, of Basel, discovered a mutation of the housefly that has a double-mutation: the animals are almost blind and cannot fly with their rolled-up wings. Dr. Bretz cross-bred them so that they became almost infertile and they entered into the trade as "Terfly." Occasionally, they are also called "flightless African houseflies."

Fannia canicularis (Fig. 54): The little housefly is at 4-5 mm a smaller version of the housefly. During summer, it can often be found in apartments. There it circles around ceiling lights instead of tree tops, around which it flies outdoors.

From the transparent, about 0.7 mm long, flattened eggs hatch strange looking maggots (Fig. 54b). They are of a dirt-yellow color; the flattened body has rows

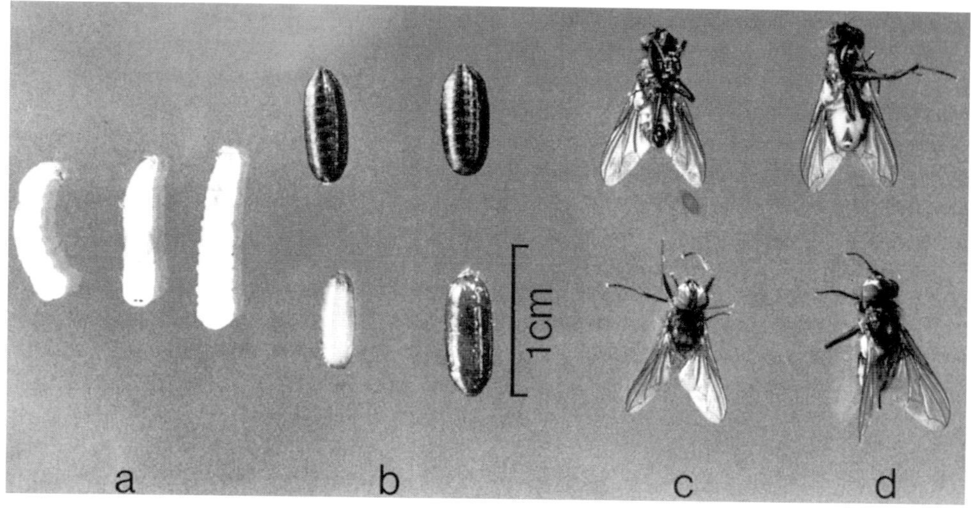

Fig. 53 Housefly (*Musca domestica*). a) Maggots, b) pupae, c) males, d) females.

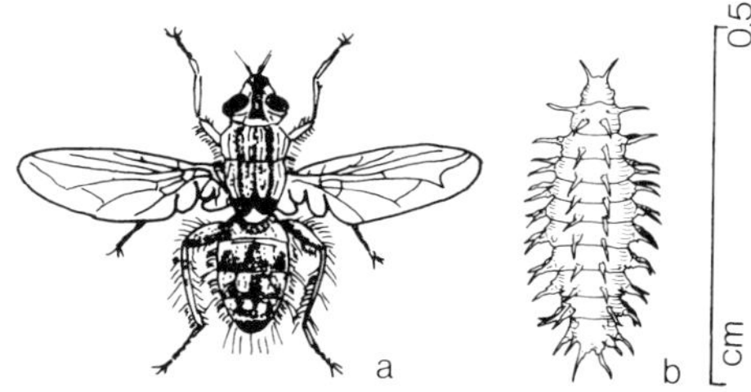

Fig. 54 Little housefly (*Fannia canicularis*). a) Fly, b) maggot.

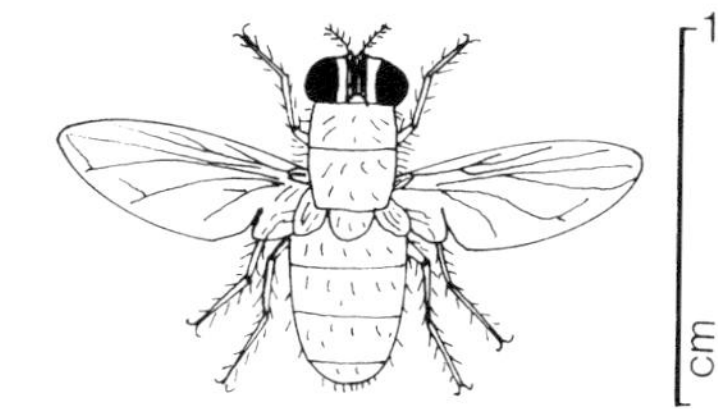

Fig. 55 Green bottle fly (*Lucilia caesar*).

of bristly appendages on the sides and on the back. The maggot grows to 5 mm, then pupates. The 4 mm long pupa is only different from the maggot in that it does not move, shows somewhat shorter appendages, and changes to a dark-brown to black color.

Calliphora erythrocephala: The large, 10-14 mm long, blowfly with its steel-blue abdomen and red cheeks that are covered with black hairs should be known to anyone, since they tend to bask on the walls of house in the early days of spring. A female can deposit eggs in packets of 10-15 eggs with a telescope-like, extensible ovipositor, a total of about 300. From them about 1.2 mm long white maggots of almost the same size hatch. When they reach 15-16 mm, they turn into 14 mm long pupae.

Lucilia caesar (Fig 55): The green bottle fly reaches a length of 8-12 mm. The thorax and the abdomen shine green to purple and appear to be dusted with gold.

134

They lay their 1 mm long eggs into meat, preferably open wounds. The maggots eat the damaged tissue. It may sound surprising that this can be quite beneficial. It prevents infections from taking hold and cleans up existing infections. Already in the 16th century the cleansing effect of maggots was discovered. But only in the 1930s of the 20th century was an explanation was found. The primary reason found was that a large number of bacteria are killed by certain biochemical processes while the maggots are eating. In addition to the maggots of the blowfly, some other species also have this capability.

The 16-17-mm-long maggots pupate into 10-11 mm long pupae.

Sarcophaga spec. (Fig. 56): Unfortunately, we could not determine the species of the flesh fly that we raised a few years ago and on which our description is based. Only specialists can tell the species apart since they look very similar. Some of the maggots live as parasites, for example those of *Sarcophaga carnaria* in earthworms, some live in carcasses or fecal matter.

Flesh flies are at a length of 15-18 mm the most impressive of all the flies discussed in this book. The upper side of the thorax is striped light gray and black; the abdomen is marked with light and dark gray spots in a chessboard pattern. The eyes are brick red. The flesh fly gives birth to live maggots; that is, the about 1.4 mm long maggots hatch inside their mother's body. The maggots grow to a size of 20 mm; the pupae are about 15-16 mm long.

Development Times: The development times for the flies are primarily determined by the length of their larval state. This depends not only on the temperature but

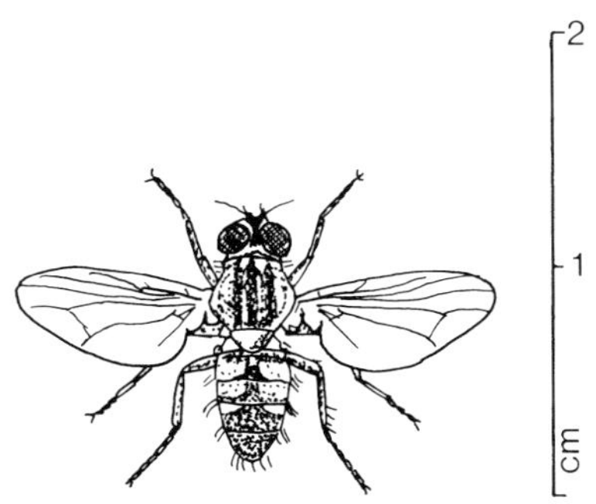

Fig. 56 Flesh fly (*Sarcophaga* spec.)

also on the quality and quantity of food available, so that values can vary considerably.

Musca domestica: The housefly reaches sexual maturity 2-3 days after hatching. It can live up to 30 days; at cooler temperatures even up to 3 months; in breeding setups the flies usually die after about 3 weeks. During this time the females lays 800-1500 eggs in batches of about 100. The Terflies, laying only 500 eggs, are considerably less productive (de Batist, 1991). The larvae hatch after 1-3 days, pupate after 8-10 days, and rest for 6-8 days until the flies hatch. The shortest times are for temperatures of 24-25°C , the longer ones for 20°C. Every 15-23 days a new generation can be expected.

Fannia canicularis: The total development time for the blowfly is about 1 month. The animals reach sexual maturity after 5-6 days; about 4-5 days after mating they lay their first eggs. The maggots, which hatch after 1-2 days, usually pupate as soon as 10-12 days later. After 8-12 days the flies hatch.

Lucilia caesar: The green bottle flies develop in a hurry. On the 2nd day of life they mate, on the 3rd day the female lays the first eggs. The maggots often crawl out of the eggs on the same day; with a good food supply they pupate in 6-7 days. The pupae rest for 5-6 days. After 11-14 days the new generation has already grown up! Breeding is most successful at 24-26°C. During her 3-4 weeks of life the green bottle fly female deposits up to 1000 eggs. *Sarcophaga* spec.: The female of the flesh fly births the first maggots 2-3 days after mating. They pupate after 8-10 days; 6-8 days later the flies hatch. The expected development time is thus 14-18 days. Each birth produces about 15-20 larvae up to a total of 600-1200 in 6 weeks.

Containers, Substrate, and Equipment: Flies require for their well-being a container that receives light and that allows them to fly around. For a small number of animals a volume of at least 3 l is necessary, for the larger species 5-6 l. The container must consist at least partially of glass, Plexiglas, transparent plastic, or gauze.

To breed a small number of flies, large pickle or pickling jars can be used, which are sealed off with a piece of nylon stocking.

The next level up are medium-sized plastic aquariums (7-15 l) that are put on the shortest side. The body part of a pair of nylon stockings can be pulled over the opening as a convenient cover: the stockings are cut off at about the middle of the legs; the leg sections serve as tunnels. For large breeding endeavors, such jars and aquariums are of course too small. We have developed breeding and hatching cages made of PVC for this purpose. Unfortunately, they are not commercially available anymore. A variety of manufacturers makes glass cages available. The

included drawings of the PVC cages might inspire do-it-yourselfers. The breeding cage (Fig. 57), which can for example be built with measurements of 30 x 25 x 35 cm and 40 x 30 x 45 cm, uses a 10 cm tall drawer in the bottom, which contains the can for egg laying, the drinking water, and the food bowl. A sliding panel can be inserted above the drawer to separate it from the flying space when the contents need to be manipulated. The front of the cage consists of glass; the lid is removable and covered with fine gauze.

The hatching cage (Fig. 58), for example 35 x 20 x 35 cm in size, has a special lid with an opening that can be closed with a sliding panel. A PVC container is also fitted with a sliding lid and fits tightly onto the opening in the box lid so that flies can be removed easily and securely.

A simpler version of this cage can easily be built. A larger Plexiglas aquarium is fitted with a wooden lid. Half the lid is covered with gauze for ventilation. In the other half a hole is cut that can be covered with a glass or other container. A piece of metal, between wooden guides, makes for a tightly fitting lid. To use this container for breeding, a round 13-14 cm hole needs to be cut in the side of the aquarium. The hole must be big enough that the cans for egg laying can be moved through it comfortably. A flexible stocking-tube is attached from the inside with tape or something similar. This hatch allows secure working inside the container. Egg-laying containers can be made from 10 x 10 x 8 cm freezer boxes or similar containers. The best substrates are sawdust or wood shavings; they remain lose, absorb moisture and store it, and are free of poisons and pests.

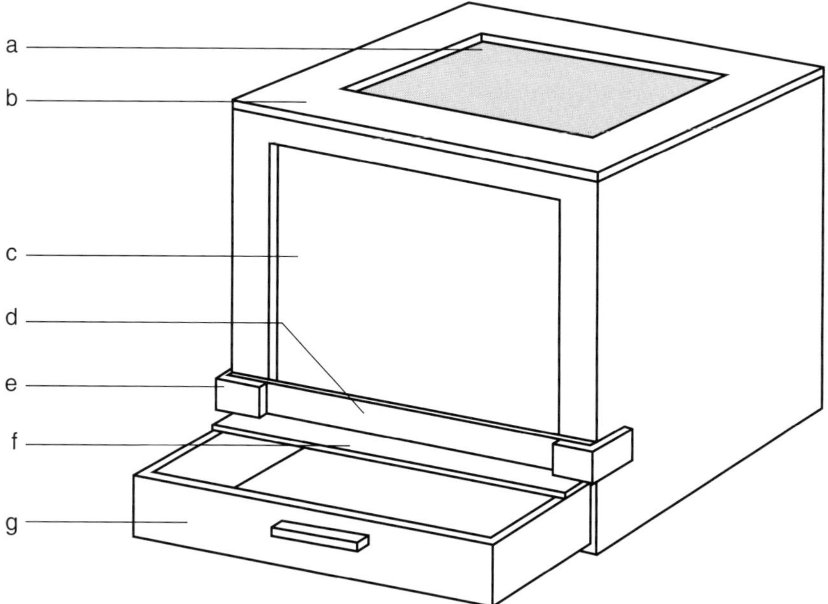

Fig. 57 Fly breeding cage made of PVC. a) Gauze, b) lid, c) glass panel, d) sliding panel, e) guiding rail, f) sliding false bottom, g) drawer.

Drinking water must not be offered from an open bowl since the flies would drown in it. A wet piece of foam can be fitted into a bird waterer.

Since flies can hold on to smooth surfaces, no other perching implements need to be provided. However, if the cage is stocked heavily, it is recommended anyway. During setup, an egg carton can be placed inside, or even a wad of paper, which Terflies absolutely need.

Food: Often the recommended food for flies has been mashed banana and vitaminized sugar water. Fed like this, the animals live only about 8-12 days, and they lay few eggs since the required proteins and minerals are missing in their diet. According to our experiences, mixtures made of milk pudding with fruit, multivita-min syrup for children, as well as honey are best for all flies. If the relatively expensive vitamin syrup is omitted, it is recommended to add codfish oil and a multivitamin powder.

All discussed species of flies, except for the housefly, require honey since in the outdoors they like to visit flowers.

If only a few flies are bred, it might be more practical to make the necessary amounts of food every time. For large-scale efforts it is useful to prepare large amounts of food ahead of time.

The following mixture is accepted by all species: Pour the contents of a 200 g package of milk pudding into a blender, add ¾ l lukewarm water, 6 Tbl. honey, 2 Tbl. codfish oil, and 1 Tbl. vitamin powder. Blend for 5 minutes.

The correct consistency for the mixture is hard to describe; it should be between barely liquid and almost liquid. This food can be stored in the refrigerator at 5°C in a bottle that is well sealed. Other ratios for the ingredients can be used depending on what the flies prefer.

Since flies can turn dry food liquid with their saliva, the ingredients can also be offered separately; a wet watering sponge plus a bowlof milk pudding and dried up cane sugar syrup, springled with vitamin powder.

Maggots: Feeding the maggots of all five species of flies on fresh meat until they pupate is without doubt the fastest and most productive methods. Ground meat that can be frozen in small portions is especially suitable. However, the blowflies, the flesh flies, and the little housefly prefer slightly rotting meat. The odors, which are intensified by the ammonia smell from the maggot excrements, prevent or at least strongly limit keeping them in rooms inhabited by humans.

For this reason, a large number of substitute foods have been tried. The little housefly and the housefly, which is probably the most important food fly, can fortunately also be bred more or less successfully with some other foods: bran with quark or milk and cocoa powder mixed up, pureed fruit, semolina mush

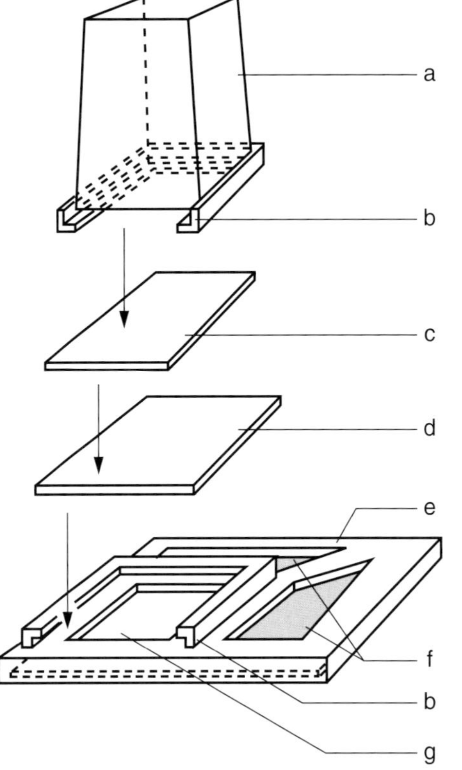

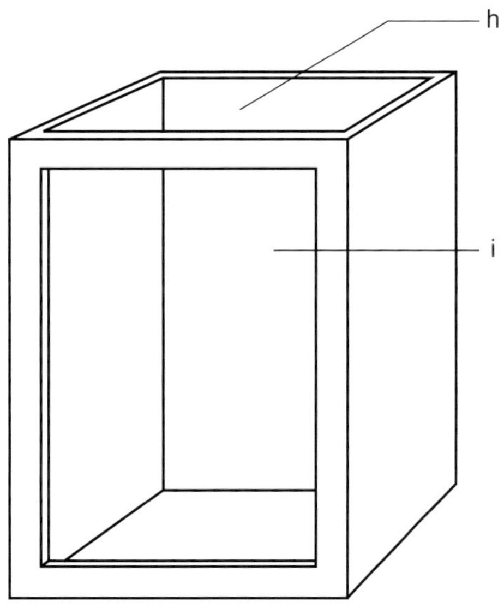

Fig. 58 Hatching cage for flies made from PVC with container for capturing them. a) Fly-catching container, b) guide rail, c) sliding panel for container, d) sliding panel for lid, e) lid, f) gauze, g) opening in lid, h) opening for hatching container, i) glass panel.

with mashed bananas or apples, softened
mouse pellet food, canned dog or cat food.
Even then, it is not always possible to
keep the cages odor free. Quark will soon
smell like rotten eggs. The bothersome
ammonia smell can vary in intensity. Fish
should never be fed since the stench is
unbearable.

We also tried some types of softened dog
kibbles. The flies willingly laid their eggs
into them, but the maggots crawled away.
It is possible that the dry food was prepared with a chemical that the maggots
cannot tolerate. Vivarium enthusiasts have
tried over and over to find ways to breed
flies odor-free. In recent times one method
that was developed by Bartholdi (1966),
and refined by Stettler (1979) and
Mudrack (1979), has been gaining popularity. According to Mudrack a transparent
freezer box measuring 20 x 10 x 8 cm is
filled with 6 cm of wheat bran. In a bowl
or measuring cup a piece of fresh baking
yeast the size of a hazelnut is dissolved in
4 Tbl. of canned milk and 4 Tbl. sugar by
adding enough warm water to yield 3/8 l
of liquid. The measured bran is added and
all is kneaded until a crumbly, slightly
moist dough forms; it must not be mushy.
The mixture is poured into the freezer
container and pressed down lightly so that
no empty spaces remain. In this cultivation medium, which is kept moist by
occasional misting, the houseflies will lay
their eggs. The maggots get additional
feedings of milk powder and yeast and
protein flakes after a few days.

This method only works when large
numbers—in the described recipe 4000-
6000—maggots constantly dig through the
medium. If there are not enough maggots,
the medium will harden, develop a crust,

and get moldy quickly and the maggots
will die.

To breed only a few animals, we recommend a method where the amount of food
is adjusted to the number of maggots. A
while ago, we tried a recipe that has
proven useful: 4 parts oats, 4 parts soy
flour, 4 parts milk powder, and 1 part
brewer's yeast are mixed dry and moistened with small amounts of water. This
food mixture remains free of odors and the
smell of ammonia develops minimally. It is
important that the maggots live in a large
amount of sawdust.

For the two species of the family Calliphoridae another cultivation medium
should be mentioned; it makes for comfortable breeding and was developed by
the Zoological Institute of the University
of Greifswald (Berndt, 1969). According
to them, one mixes 180 g wheat bran with
90 g sawdust, 405 ml blood, and 4.5 g
fresh yeast. For his daily use, Berndt uses
equal volumes of coarse wheat bran,
defibrinated beef blood, and sifted, fresh
sawdust from leafy trees. For 200 larvae
50 cm^2 of medium are required.

Breeding Conditions:

Light: Even though the flies can be bred in
complete darkness for many generations, it
is more natural to make some light
available for 8-12 hours daily since these
animals are diurnal. If the breeding cage
is not in a bright room, incandescent and
fluorescent light bulbs are suitable sources
of light. They are installed above the
container as they get dirty too quickly if
installed inside.

Temperature: A room temperature of 19-
21°C is sufficient for breeding flies if no
fast development times are required.
Otherwise, the temperature must be 24-

28°C. Terflies require more heat than ordinary houseflies; below 22°C they reproduce poorly. The best sources of heat are incandescent light bulbs and infrared heat emitters. If heat is provided from below, for example, with a heating pad, the water and egg-laying containers may dry out too fast. Maggots require no additional heat since at a sufficient population density they will generate their own heat that can exceed 30°C.

Humidity: The relative air humidity can range widely from 25-70%. If the offered food is rather liquid and always available, the flies may not require drinking water, provided they are kept at a temperature of about 20°C. It is safer to always have drinking water available. At the higher temperatures the little houseflies, blow-flies, and flesh flies must have a sponge with water available daily.

Eggs, maggots, and pupae require some moisture. Their substrate must never dry out but should not be soggy either.

Notes: Since small and large-scale setups are operated in basically the same manner, no distinction needs to be made in the following notes.

Breeding flies is a topic with many variations. The beginner often does not know where to start. This is why we will give a detailed description here.

When starting to breed, two paths can be chosen. In the first one, one container always holds always a certain number of breeding flies that are regularly replaced by newly hatched animals, and another container holds the flies used for food. For the second method there is no such separation, and the number of flies is influenced by making substrate for egg laying available more or less often. Young flies will replace the old ones soon enough. If certain amounts of flies are needed regularly, the first method is definitely more practical.

To breed flies with little odor is a big effort that requires a meticulous schedule. This is especially true for small setups, which are often kept in living spaces. The following paragraphs describe the tasks for a breeding setup according to the first method. A bowl of water is added to a prepared breeding container. Then, depending on your requirements, 25-150 pairs of flies are added, which must be fed immediately. A small amount of food puree is smeared on the gauze in the lid so that nothing drips through. The flies will eat the food without getting stuck or drowning. The amount should be measured such that no food is left after a day. The food must be replenished daily. If the food is filled about 0.5 cm high into a dish and placed inside the cage, food to last for 2-3 days can be offered. In this case, the paste should of a thicker consistency. In spite of this, some animals will fall into this "swamp" and will be unable to get out.

Once the females carry eggs, about 4-10 days after hatching depending on the species, the egg-laying container is placed inside the cage. The freezer box is filled loosely with moist wood shavings; a small amount of food is buried in the substrate as an incentive for laying eggs and as a first food for the maggots.

A pea-or hazelnut-sized piece of meat is irresistible to all flies. The houseflies will even lay their eggs on wet paper. Since the flesh flies will deliver maggots, they ought to be given additional meat.

After 1-3 days the egg-laying container is removed; it should contain plenty of eggs and larvae. It depends on how many flies are needed whether a new egg-laying container is provided immediately or a few days later.

The full egg-laying container is placed into a larger jar or bowl and covered tightly with a piece of stocking or gauze, since especially the green bottle and blow fly maggots will climb out of their container if the temperature is over 30°C and there is not enough food.

From now on the maggots must be inspected twice daily to make sure they have enough but not too much food. Meat in particular should be consumed within 24 hours so that no rot and odors of decay develop. Only fresh meat should be used. About 1-2 days after the egg-laying container has been removed from the breeding cage, all the larvae should have hatched. The contents of the egg-laying container are dumped into another container and moist wood shavings are added to double or triple the amount of substrate. This gives the fast-growing maggots sufficient space to develop.

No matter what the maggots are fed, the ammonia odor cannot be prevented, only limited. If the maggots are raised on meat, they must be separated from their wood shavings every day. If a mixture of oats, soy four, milk powder, and brewer's yeast is used, it depends on the number of maggots whether it will be necessary to sift the substrate once or twice or never during development. When following Mudrack's (1979) instructions, the maggots and pupae remain in the bran until the flies hatch.

As long as the larvae are relatively small, they can be rinsed together with the wood shavings. Their container is filled with lukewarm water, everything is poured into a fine-meshed sieve and rinsed with water for a short time. After the water has drained well, the maggots and wood shavings are dumped into a clean container and fresh wood shavings are added until the desired level of moisture is reached. Then they must be fed immediately.

For maggots of any size, a piece of coarse fabric (potato bag, floor rag) is best suited as a "sieve." The fabric is stretched over a wooden frame or a bucket that had its bottom removed. It is important that the catch container is a little larger than the sifting frame that can be put directly over the fresh wood shavings. The substrate with the maggots is distributed on the fabric in thin layers and illuminated from above. The maggots will squeeze down and through the fabric and fall into the fresh substrate.

If the larvae are restless even if there is plenty of food available, it means that they will pupate within a day or two. The green bottle maggots will also crawl up the sides of the jar and squeeze in between the jar, the stocking, and the rubber bands so that different containers that can be sealed better must be used. If necessary, the maggots can be strained through the fabric sieve once more into dry wood shavings. Be careful since wet maggots will climb any wall up to 1 m tall! A rim of Vaseline might help keep them from escaping. As soon as the maggots pupate, the wood shavings should be lightly moistened. The pupae must not dry out or no flies will hatch. They require at least 80% relative air humidity or otherwise should be misted occasionally.

It will take a few days for the flies to emerge from their pupae. During this time the pupae can be moved into the fly cage or to another jar. Any jar or bowl can also be sealed with a stocking and the flies are be transferred after they hatch.

If the maggots are not fed often enough or if they do not receive food after they reach a certain size, they will pupate early. The resulting flies will of course be smaller than normal. Such forced pupation can be induced deliberately for houseflies if a food size between fruit flies and houseflies is required for raising frogs or lizards, and one does not want to also breed *Fannia*. Once the maggots are about 6-7 mm long, feeding is halted. At about 27°C they will pupate quickly. Of course, fully developed normal-sized houseflies should always be produced as breeding stock since they are much more productive egg layers.

The flightless and blind houseflies require their own breeding methodologies that compensate for their handicaps. De Batist (1991) has described this in detail. Dieter Bretz told us about his proven method: A ½ l (2 cup) polyethylene container is filled to ¾ with wheat bran that has been moistened with pasteurized whole milk so that the bran gets lumpy but is not wet. A pinch of vitamin A, ½ pinch of Nipagin, and ½ cube of fresh baking yeast have been stirred into the milk previously. A sugar cube is placed on top of the bran mixture, and a generous teaspoon full of ready-to-hatch pupae are placed in a corner. The jar is covered with kitchen towels that are fastened with a rubber band. That's all the work! If everything goes according to plan, after 14 days (at 25°C the pupae of the next generation will be in the jar. The jar is filled with water, a few drops of dishwashing liquid are added, stirred, and left to sit for ½ hour. Then the water is poured over a kitchen sieve and

the contents rinsed. The contents of the sieve are dumped into a bowl with much water; 1 tablespoon of salt is dissolved per liter of water, everything is stirred together, and left to stand for another half hour until the pupae can be skimmed off the surface.

Every few generations the flies that are to become breeding stock should be inspected. Over time the rolled up wing mutation will disappear or the mutated flies managed to mate with normal ones; only mutated flies should be chosen for breeding stock

The bottom of the container for the flies to be used as food animals is covered with wads of paper and the flies receive a liquid food, vitamin-fortified milk (A and B without B_{12}) on paper towels. Terflies will drown in open dishes.

All good things rarely come in the same package. You will have to choose between normal houseflies and Terflies. The normal ones are easy to breed and handle. However, it is impossible to let them lose in the terrarium without at least some escapees. For frogs, which live on the bottom, most flies remain unreachable since they congregate under the lid of the terrarium. This does not happen with Terflies. On the other hand, they are not as productive and are less tolerant of mistakes.

Storage: The maggots of all flies can be stored at 2-5°C for up to 6 weeks. The pupae of the housefly can be kept for at most 6 weeks at 2-5°C, those of the green bottle and blow flies at 5°C for over 8 weeks. Wood shavings should be added as maggots and pupae must not dry out.

Pests and Diseases: Unfortunately, flies are especially attracted to foul-smelling and unappetizing substances. When they sit down, they get loaded up with bacteria, worm eggs, and other disease-causing agents. Over 6 million bacteria have been counted on one single housefly! When the flies then land on our food, a number of organisms are always left behind that can be taken up by humans or animals and possibly cause diseases. This is why it is important to never let food sit out uncovered. We sincerely doubt that any wild-caught disease-carrying flies would make a good food for vivarium animals. The flies themselves suffer from a number of parasites that are inconsequential for vivarium animals. Worth mentioning is a fungus, *Empusa muscae*, that can infest all species of flies and kill them without exception. The mycelium of the fungus spreads through the whole body of the fly until it dies. The fly will sit and it will look so natural, that it appears alive, but it will be surrounded by a circle of white spores. Flies are more often affected by this fungus in fall. If one infected fly is detected, it is best to destroy the whole breeding stock since the fungus is very contagious.

Feeding: Flies are especially easy to dust with calcium and mineral powders since quite a bit of powder adheres to their many hairs and around the wings. Young lizards and salamanders should only get dusted flies. It is easiest to place the food flies directly into the terrarium—who would want to hand-feed flies? This requires a fly-proof cage. Terrariums usually fill this requirement, but not bird cages. Birds should therefore probably be fed maggots for the most part. Make sure that the maggots are torn or chewed well as their skin is very tough. Otherwise, it can happen, that the maggots are excreted whole, or in the worst case, they chew on the digestive organs of their predator. For this reason, maggots should not be fed to weak or newly acquired animals. They should only be given to fish in small numbers. When feeding flies to fish, they should be cooled so that they cannot escape. It is almost impossible to list all the animals that like to dine on flies. Among fish the dwarf cichlids should be mentioned, which do not thrive without live food; other types of fish also like flies, as for example, barbs, barbs, Panchax species, tetras, killifish, archer fish, and butterfly fish. Raising smaller and medium-sized frogs and lizards without flies is almost unthinkable; as for example, poison dart frogs, tree frogs, reed frogs, anoles, geckoes, and chameleons. Among birds tanagers, Timaliidae babblers, white-eyes, leaf birds, mockingbirds, shrikes, stilts, and warblers all love flies. Among invertebrates, the list includes praying mantids, spiders, and predatory beetles.

Advantages and Disadvantages:

Advantages:

- Favorite and excellent food for many vivarium animals
- Can be bred in unlimited numbers
- Flies are quiet and odor-free; maggots –especially of the houseflycan be kept in ways that produce little or no odor.

Disadvantages:

- Relatively large amount of work
- Large numbers of maggots can cause bothersome smells in living areas
- If the maggots are fed on meat, portions must be frozen

Butterflies (Lepidoptera)

The order of butterflies, the Lepidoptera, with about 140,000 species first brings up memories of colorful butterflies. Unfortunately, it is almost impossible to breed them and moths systematically because of the specialized feeding requirements of their caterpillars. Especially the Owlet moths (Noctuidae) with their thick bodies are ideal prey so that breeding them would be desirable.

Maybe one species will turn out to be easy to breed. One possibility is the hibernating willow moth, which lays its eggs on willow leaves, or the *Mamestra* genus, which includes the cabbage moth.

Species that go through two generations annually in temperate climates might also be suitable. In addition, some tropical butterflies with hairless caterpillars might offer possibilities. It would be necessary that the caterpillars do not eat just one food and would accept lettuce, carrots, or some other easily available food substitute in winter.

Among the small butterflies are several that are considered agricultural and forest pests. The beekeeper's dread is the vivarium enthusiast's joy: moths from the family Pyralidae eat primarily old honeycombs but will also eat bee larvae, and they cover the honeycombs with their gossamer. For the vivarium enthusiasts they provide enrichment for their animals' menu.

The biggest and most noticeable part of a butterfly is its wings, which are covered on with small scales (Squamulae) that are arranged like roof tiles on both sides. These scales determine the color and pattern of the wings. Most butterflies use their long proboscis to lick nectars and wound secreations. Their larvae, however, the caterpillars, whose abdomen has only simple extremities, have mouthparts for biting and they eat all sorts of plant parts, especially leaves, but also roots, flowers, fruit, and grains.

Greater Wax Moth (*Galleria mellonella*) Lesser Wax Moth (*Achroea grisella*)

Description: *Galleria mellonella* (Fig. 59): The large wax moth has a wingspan of 28-35 mm. At rest, the moths are about 10-14 mm long. Their base color is light gray to light yellowish, the forewings are marbled light brown. Not only the wings but also the abdomen and legs are covered with scales. The genders can be distinguished easily: the female has a longer and fatter abdomen than the male.

The 1.5 mm long caterpillars, which are often falsely called wax worms, hatch from white, 1 mm long, slim eggs. After 4 molts they reach 24-28 mm in length and about 5 mm in diameter. The red brown head is clearly set off from the dirt gray, somewhat transparent, body. To pupate the caterpillars make a cocoon. The pupa measures 8-10 mm, the cocoon about 16 mm.

Achroea grisella: With a wingspan for 16-19 mm and a body length of about 8 mm, the lesser wax moth is one of the smallest butterflies. It is well camouflaged with its dark markings on its forewings, which shine silvery. The head is light yellow and covered with hairs. In this species, too, the females have a larger abdomen.

It is amazing that the caterpillars reach a length of about 16 mm with a 3 mm diameter, since they are only 1 mm long when they hatch from the 0.8 mm eggs. The 6 mm long dark brown pupae rest in a 9 mm long cocoons.

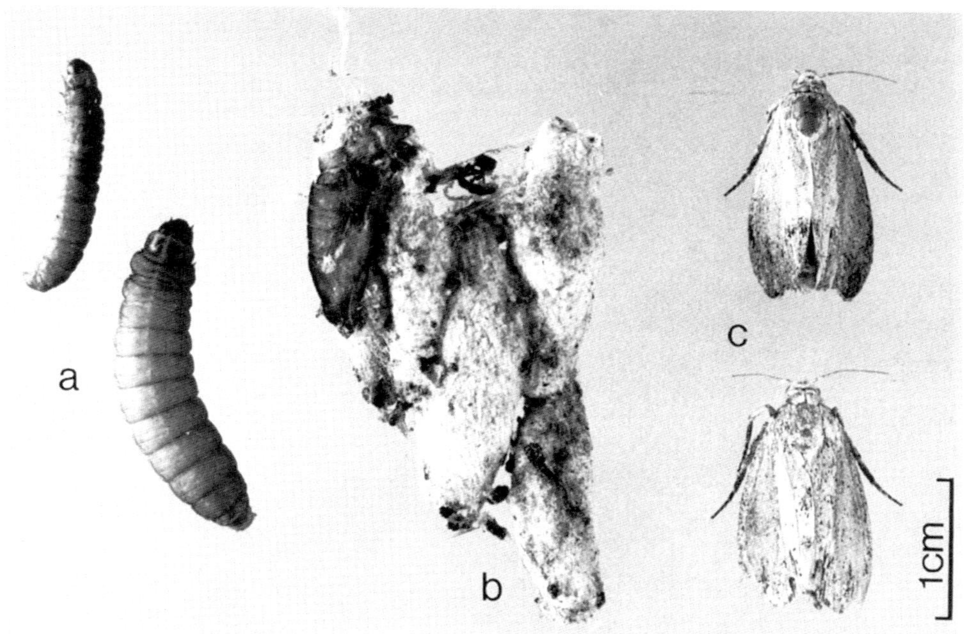

Fig. 59 Large wax moth (*Galleria mellonella*). a) Larvae, b) cocoons, c) moths.

Development Times: Since the temperature inside a beehive is around 27-28°C, this is the ideal temperature for breeding wax moths. At this temperatures the generations follow each other at intervals of 6-7½ weeks. The caterpillars hatch after 5-8 days and reach their full size in 18-25 days. Then they spin their cocoon and pupate, which takes about 2 days. The pupa rests for about 12 days. The moths start mating on the same day that they emerge and remain in their copulation position for a whole day. The female lays her first eggs 4-5 days after mating., *G. mellonella* up to 150 per clutch, but mostly 40-60, and *A. grisella* 20-50. The large wax moth can lay up to 800 eggs, the small wax moth 300.

In a beehive wax moths live up to 6 weeks, in a breeding setup at most 3 weeks, mostly only 10-14 days. This is probably because the bees offer the wax moths optimal conditions, namely even warmth and humidity and cleanliness. Therefore, in captivity, egg production remains significantly below the maximum.

If the wax moths are kept at 22-24°C, the development time extends to 10-14 days.

Containers, Cultivation Media, and Equipment: Wax moths can be bred in containers of 1-30 l, for example household plastic containers, large jars, cans, plastic buckets, small plastic aquariums, and home-built boxes made of PVC or glass (Fig. 60). Wooden containers are not suitable since the caterpillars will chew through them over time. All these containers must be

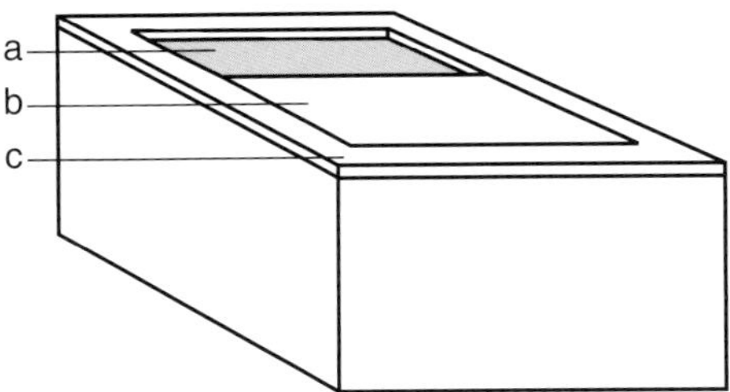

Fig. 60 Breeding cage for wax moths made from PVC. a) Fine gauze, b) glass sliding cover, c) lid.

equipped with a tightly closing lid and with at least one ventilation window that can be covered with the finest, nonrusting wire mesh of 0.4 mm mesh size. The caterpillars chew through plastic meshes, and if the mesh-size is larger, many of the freshly hatched and at first very active caterpillars will escape. For plastic containers, gauze windows can be glued to the sides, for glass jars, an opening can be cut into the lid.

The interior is taken up mostly by the food; that is the honeycombs or the food paste. A few corrugated cardboard tubes or strips of cardboard are placed vertically since the caterpillars like to pupate on them as well as on the sides and under the lid. Since wax moths prefer warmth and darkness, it may be advantageous to create a small breeding chamber for them. A wooden cabinet as described on page 23 can be used. Wax moths can also be housed in a dark boiler room.

Food: Wax moths feed, as their name indicates on wax, in particular old, dirty honeycombs. If you get lucky, you might find an understanding beekeeper who will provide the necessary supply. The honeycombs should be frozen for several days to prevent uninvited guests from getting into the breeding setup. Soon it will become obvious that acquiring the food can be quite expensive in the long run. There have, therefore, been many attempts to get wax moths used to eating an artificial diet. The so-called Haydak-medium was the best known artificial medium for a long time, a moist dough made of 600 g flour, 200 g low-fat milk powder, 200 g wheat bran, 100 g dry yeast, 550 g honey and 550 g glycerin.

A newer mixture, which has been used successfully and which results in about the same development times as feeding honeycombs, has the following ingredients:

  500 g liquid honey (warmed to 35°C)
  500 g glycerin (available from drugstores or pharmacies)
  200 g brewer's yeast
  200 g wheat germ
  200 g low-fat milk powder
  2 kg what bran; or 1.5 kg wheat bran with 500 g oats

The honey and glycerin are mixed thoroughly by hand or with a blender. The dry ingredients are stirred together and slowly added to the honey-glycerin mixture. The resulting mass is stirred and kneaded until it becomes a sticky, shiny dough that is moist and crumbly and smells of bee wax. This food can be stored in the refrigerator for several months and even longer in the freezer. After freezing or refrigerating, the mixture should be stored for several days at 30°C so that the honey liquefies, since the caterpillars will not eat crystallized honey. To start a breeding container, this mixture is added to the breeding container to about 4 cm and a few corrugated cardboard tubes are stuck into it vertically.

Breeding Conditions:

Light: Considering that it is pitch dark

inside a beehive, it makes sense that wax moths avoid light. Jars are practical for breeding because they are easy to check, but they must be put in a dark place.

Temperature: As already mentioned, the bees try to keep the temperature inside their hive at 27-28°C. This is the optimal breeding temperature. At 22-24°C reproduction is satisfactory, but temperatures above 34°C must be avoided. Note that if the breeding containers are stocked heavily, the caterpillars will produce heat on their own, which will raise the temperature by 2-4 degrees above the ambient temperature.

Humidity: Wax moths tolerate neither wetness nor high humidity. No condensation must be allowed to form on the sides of the container. This is why two ventilation openings are recommended.

Notes: Wax moths have been captive-bred for over 40 years. This proves that breeding can be done successfully without too many tricks and special difficulties. The biggest problem used to be acquiring old honeycombs. With the availability of an artificial food, some independence has been created in this matter, and the popularity of wax moths should only increase.

Small-scale breeding: Containers of 1-5 l volume are well suited for small setups. As with all breeding endeavors, it is advantageous to work them on a schedule. Setting up 2-3 containers over specific periods of time guarantees a steady supply of wax worms.

For a 2 l jar about 30-40 moths, cocoons, or large caterpillars of the little wax moth, or 20 of the large wax moth are a good starting number. From this starting stock, about 300 caterpillars can be expected. Of course, a certain percentage must be allowed to pupate so that breeding can continue.

The moths require flying space to mate. This is why the breeding container should only be filled halfway with honeycombs or to 4 cm with the artificial food. This is probably the right amount of food for the caterpillars. If they become restless, food must be added immediately; if they are left to fast for more than two days, the caterpillars will pupate early. However, the adult caterpillars will also wander around looking for a place for their cocoon.

Large-scale breeding: For a large-scale endeavor breeding containers are also set up in regular intervals. The difference is that larger containers of 5-30 l are used, and possibly several at each stage. The breeding stock consists of 60-150 moths; a large PVC container can hold up to 1000 moths and 3000 caterpillars.

As for all large-scale breeding, a separate room is recommended, which can be heated to the desired temperature.

Storage: Wax moths cannot be bred ahead of time since they do not store well. When put into the refrigerator, the caterpillars will die, and the moths survive only a few days. The only possible measure is to allow the temperature to drop to 20°C to slow development.

Pests and Diseases: When the air humidity is high, the feces of the caterpillars get moldy very easily. If the caterpillars walk through moist or moldy feces, they die. Good ventilation of the breeding containers is therefore essential.

Ichneumon wasps, which lay their eggs into caterpillars one at a time are rarely seen if the containers are stored tightly closed.

Unfortunately, the wax moth setups are susceptible to mites. If only a few of them are seen, they can be baited with grease. If there is a massive infestation, the stock must be destroyed, all containers cleaned with hot or boiling water, and the space, where the setup stood, must be wiped and cleaned thoroughly. No new setup should be placed in the same location for several weeks.

Feeding: Caterpillars that are ready to pupate are easiest to remove as they crawl out of the honeycombs or the cultivation medium; they can simply be collected. If smaller caterpillars are needed, the honey-combs or the artificial food must be taken apart and searched for the desired speci-mens. Since the caterpillars shy away from light and hide quickly at the slightest dis-turbance, one is forced to work in the dark. The caterpillars are offered to all vivarium animals, except fish, in a bowl with smooth sides and a curled rim, or directly from a needle. The moths are rather lazy but can fly up unexpectedly. A well-stocked cage should not be opened—nobody can catch this many moths!

To feed large numbers of moths, smaller jars can be used for breeding, or a number of grown up caterpillars or pupae are moved into a separate smaller container. This container is then set into the ter-rarium and opened. Tapping the jar will scare the moths and they will fly up.

A breeding cage can also be put into the refrigerator for a short time. The cold and quiet moths are easier to handle.

The PVC container should have a sliding door in the lid. If a container is placed on top of the opening, the moths fly into it and they can then be used for food. Caterpillars and moths, which taste of honey, are a favorite food for most vivarium animals. For killifish, cichlids and tetras, they are a festive dinner. Frogs and smaller lizards, like geckos and agamas, skinks, and many chameleons will devour the caterpillars excitedly, and the moths too. Wax worms are essential for feeding insect-eating birds; many small mammals, as for example, marmoset monkeys, bush babies, and slow loris will go wild about them.

Even though wax worms are favored, they should not be fed in large amounts or exclusively since they are very fatty. Their fat content is at about 19% in fresh weight, which is significantly higher than meal-worms.

Advantages and Disadvantages:
Advantages:
- Small amount of work
- Highly nutritious food animal
- No odor
- Relatively short development time
- Does not reproduce in apartments/ houses
- Food can be prepared ahead of time

Disadvantages:
- Breeding setups get easily infested with mites
- Escaped large caterpillars can eat holes into books or padded furniture to pupate inside

Mammals

Among vertebrates, there are a large number of valuable food animals, but they require a significant investment in time and effort to breed. For several reasons, the selection here is limited to two species: mice and rats. They belong to the family Muridae, the mouse-like, within the order

Rodentia (rodents). This order comprises almost half of all mammals. As food animals, variations of the house mouse (*Mus m. musculus*) are best known and they reproduce fastest. The African soft-furred rat (*Mastomys natalensis*; often still known under its old name *M. coucha*) is less odorous, but bites so much that it is risky to feed specimens to, for example, smaller snakes. Care must also be taken when handling this species. The desert mice of the species *Meriones*, which belong to the hamsters and do not smell when kept clean, are also easy to keep. However, they are very cute animals and many vivarium enthusiasts will find it difficult to use them as food.

While mice appear cute occasionally, rats are rather despised even though they are smart animals that are indispensable as lab and food animals.

House Mouse
(*Mus musculus musculus*)
Norway Rat
(*Rattus norvegicus*)

Description: *Mice* (Fig. 61): At a total length of 15-19 cm, half of which is tail, the house mice reach a weight of 40-60 g; the females are somewhat heavier. The ears and tail are hairless. The fur is usually of one color, sometimes spotted. Best known is the white mouse, but brown and black mice have been bred, and many other color variations including milk-coffee brown, blue gray, cinnamon, and silver white.
In adults, the gender is easy to distinguish: the females have teats, the males testicles. Depending on the size of the litter and the variety, the young weigh between 1.0-1.7 g and measure 3.2-3.6 cm without their tale,

which is about the same size as an adult black cricket.
Rats (Fig. 62): The Norway rat (*Rattus norvegicus*) forms the basis of all labora-tory and feeder rats. Albinos are bred most frequently, but colored and patterned strains are also available.
About half of the body length is taken up by the hairless tail; the animals reach a total length of 40-47 cm. The males are heavier than the females; they weigh depending on race 500-700 g, the females 400-500 g. The adult male can easily be distinguished from the female by its testicles.
Newborn rats weigh 4-6 g and measure 4-5 cm not counting the tail.

Development Times: *Mice*: Mice reach sexual maturity at the age of 4-6 weeks, but they should not be bred until they are 7-8 weeks old. After 18-24 days the female gives birth to 1-18 young, 9-15 in average, and nurses them for 4 weeks. Already after 2½-3 weeks, at the latest on the 21st day, the young should be separated from the adults and also by gender. On one hand, the female is expected to give birth again soon, and on the other hand, an early, uncontrolled mating of the young should be prevented. At this age the genders may be difficult to tell apart. The males can be determined easier by lifting the skin of the belly at the rear part of the abdomen with thumb and forefinger, which will move the testicles into the scrotum.
The young mice are fully furred at 8-10 days and weigh 5-7 g. After 2 weeks they open their eyes, leave the nest for the first time, accept solid food, and produce normal feces. At 16 days they reach their skittish age; they jump at the smallest disturbance and escape easily if the cage is

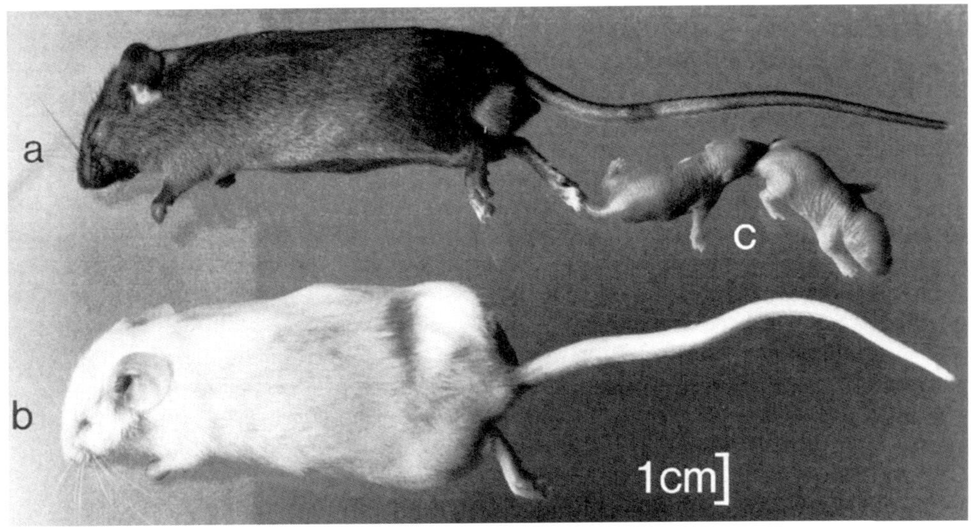

Fig. 61 Mouse (*Mus musculus musculus*). a) Male, b) females, c) young.

not completely sealed. On average, the mice weigh 10-12 g at 20 days and 15-19 g at 30 days age.

Depending on the breeding stock, the adult mice live from 1-3½ years. They are useful for breeding for about one year; a female can produce 100-135 young in that time.

Rats: Rats reach sexual maturity at an age of 5-9 weeks; they should however not be bred until they are fully grown at about 12 weeks age, otherwise the females will eat up their first two litters. After a pregnancy of 3 weeks the female gives birth to 9-12, sometimes up to 23, young and nurses them for 4 weeks. This time extends to 5 weeks if the female is at the same time nursing a large litter. For large litters, the young should be separated after 4 weeks, for normal-sized litters after 3 weeks. Young animals of the same age can be sexed by the size of their genitals and their distance to the anus: both are larger in males. A second method is described in the section on mice.

At 10 days age the young rats have quadrupled their birth weight of about 5 g. After 20 days they weigh 40-50 g, after 50 days 120-155 g, and after 80 days 175-240 g. Males grow faster and weigh 12% more than females after 100 days. At the age of 10-17 days the young open their eyes, eat solid food for the first time 3-4 days later, and are fully furred after 14 days.

After a year, but at the latest after 15 months, the breeding stock should be replaced with younger animals. A female has raised 100-120 young by that time. Rats reach an age of 3 years, 7 years in exceptional cases.

Container, Substrate, and Equipment:
Mice: Specially developed plastic tubs made of Makrolon polycarbonate plastic with wire-mesh lids are extremely suitable breeding containers for mice (Fig. 63). These cages are easy to sterilize, can be stacked without the lid, and are almost

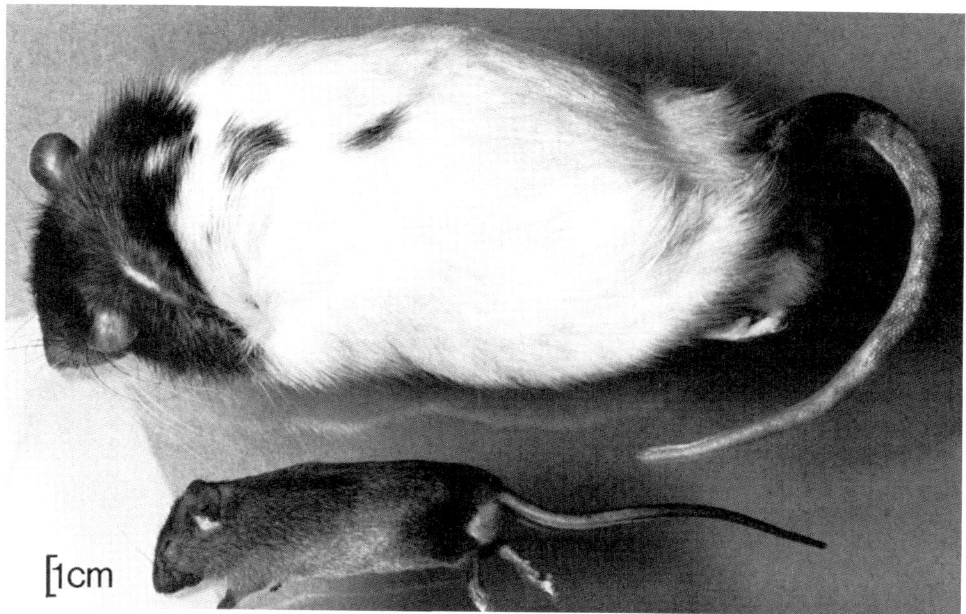

Fig. 62 Top: Male rat (*Rattus norvegicus*), bottom: male mouse (*mus musculus musculus*).

indestructible. Indentations in the lid accept the water bottle and the food so that it is rarely necessary to open the cage. These cages are available in a number of sizes. For a few years such cages have also been produced from other plastics at a lower price. Our experience is that they are not as durable.

To keep only a few animals, glass tanks, which can be homemade, can be used if the glass panels are glued together with aquarium-safe silicon glue. For better ventilation, the upper half of one side panel should be made of wire mesh. Wood, just like plastic, holds heat well, so that for cool locations or rooms where temperature varies a lot, it is the recommended building material. Mice chew, so that only hard woods like teak, beech, or oak can be used. The boards should be at least 13 mm thick,

and the bottom can be reinforced with a plastic insert.

Wire cages should only be used in rooms that are uniformly heated. The temperature should be regulated with a thermostat. Chrome plated metal will rust after a short time because of the uric acid, therefore high-grade steel should be used.

The height of the cages should be 15 cm, better 20 cm so that the jumpy hoppers cannot escape. The required floor space depends on the number of animals. A breeding group of 1 male, 7-8 females, and their young require 1500 cm^2 until they are separated, that is for example a cage of 50 x 30 cm. For a 1:4 breeding group an area of 40 x 25 cm is required, for a 2:15 group a cage size of 60 x 40 cm, for one female with young a 20 x 20 cm cage, and for ten youngsters a container that measures

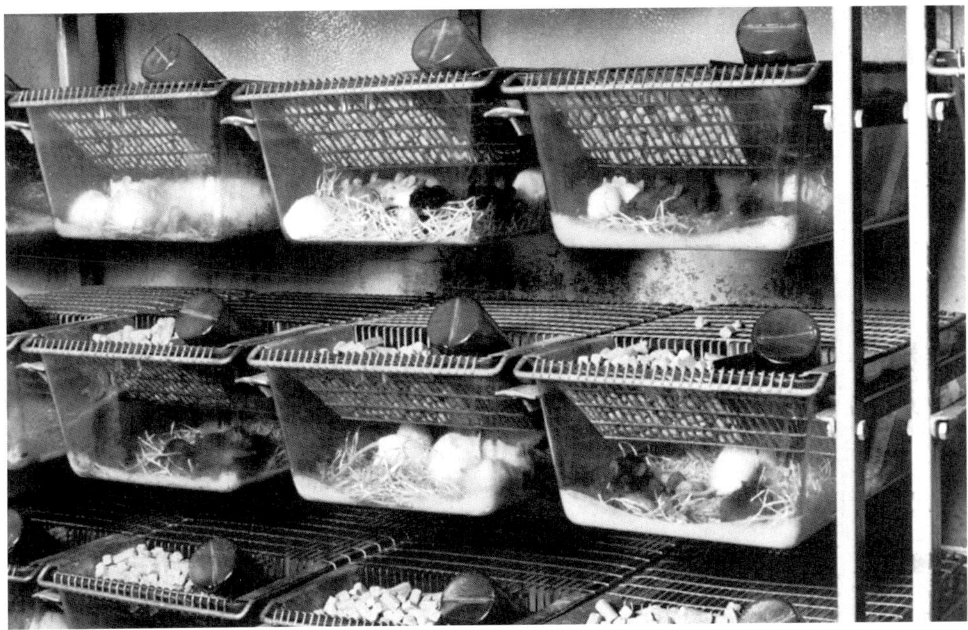

Fig. 63 Breeding mice in plastic tubs.

30 x 20 cm.
Mice like to move around a lot, so the cages should not be too small, even if the animals are "only" bred for food.
An exercise wheel offers additional options for activity.
Every cage needs a nesting box with a 4 cm round opening. Nesting boxes can be purchased or made from wood. Their size depends on the number of females, for example 15 x 8 x 10 cm for four females. However, the animals will chew up such a box rather efficiently, and it also offers ideal conditions for the proliferation of disease causing agents, so that it must be replaced every 6-10 weeks. For large-scale breeding the nesting box is done away with in favor of a dark corner for nesting. Sawdust, wood shavings, cellulose, or pure, sterilized peat moss are proven substrates. Sawdust is the most absorbent of these. Wood shavings from pine wood, which can be acquired from large saw-mills, crumble to dust and should not be used. To make sure no diseases are introduced, disinfected materials are used. Kitchen paper towels and fertilized peat moss are unsuitable. The absorbency rate of the substrate is extremely important. If the rather pricey Makrolon tubs are used, it is worthwhile to protect them by using a substrate that is absorbent and that is changed often. Paper and hay can be offered as nesting materials. Keeping the mice on wire racks is not recommended since the nesting material will fall through the gaps. Wire-bottom cages are only useful to hold young animals until they are used as feeders.
Offering drinking water in bowls is

152

impractical and not done anymore. The water gets dirty all the time and has to be changed daily or even more often, and it takes up valuable floor space. Drinking bottles, which are usually made of plastic, only have advantages. They are attached on the outside of the cage, above or on the side. They are closed either with a rubber stopper through which a straight or bent glass tube of about 2 mm diameter is pushed, or a metal cap with a hole about 1 mm wide, so that the mice obtain water when they lick on it.

The containers, lids, and water bottles should be disinfected about once a month. Ask the manufacturer which detergents are safe to use for your tubs. If the breeding setups are in a separate room, the room should be disinfected once a month with Aldehyde.

Rats: Since they are larger, rats require larger cages that are at least 20 cm high, preferably 25 cm, so that they can stand upright. A surface area of 40-50 x 70-80 cm is suitable for a 2:10-15 breeding group or 25-40 young rates. The nesting cage for a female should measure 40 x 25 cm. The best cages are made of Makrolon polycarbonate plastic tubs with wire lids. Unfortunately, these tubs are only available up to 20 cm height, but the available 5 cm guinea pig extensions can be used to achieve the necessary height. Since rats do not chew as much as mice, wooden cages work well, especially if only a few animals are kept. Because of the large amounts of urine produced, frequent cleaning is essential. Steal metal cages can be used in climate-controlled rooms. For large-scale breeding, cages with wire-mesh bottoms are practical; feces and urine drop into a removable tray. Such cages can be cleaned

easily. However, they are completely unsuitable for females to have their young, as they require nesting materials. For substrates the same as for mice can be used. Wood-wool is a favorite nesting material.

Food: Like all animals, mice and rats require protein (amino acids), carbohydrates, fatty acids, minerals, and vitamins in balanced amounts for a healthy metabolism. The nutritional needs of breeding animals can be met in two ways. Safe, simple, economical, and tried and proven for many years are standard food mixtures for mice and rats. These are pellets that are available in a variety of sizes. The pellets made by the Altromin company, for example, contain 23% protein, 5% fat, 4.5% fiber, 6.5% ash, 13.5% water, and 47.5% carbohydrates, a total of 12 amino acids, the minerals calcium, phosphorus, magnesium and sodium, several trace elements and the vitamins A, B_1, B_2, B_6, B_{12}, D_3, E, K_4, niacin, panthothenic acid, folic acid, biotin, and choline. According to Schmidt (1973), young rats and pregnant females require 30-40% protein. For this the second diet offered by the Altromin Company is recommended, which contains 32% protein. However, we know of many rat setups that have been fed exclusively on the standard diet without any problems.

Adult mice require 3-5 g of this food daily, nursing females more, about 6-10 g. For rats the corresponding amounts are 12-15 g and 20-40 g. Depending on the number of animals and the size of the feeding container, the food has to be replenished once or twice a week. Since this diet contains everything the animals need, only water needs to be offered in addition.

Mostly for the purpose of being comprehensive, the traditional feeding method is also described here. It requires a lot more time and consideration and is only feasible for small numbers of purchased animals. Mice are fed chicken mash, greens (lettuce, dandelion, carrots), oats, linseeds, bread soaked in milk as a treat, and a dried shrimp every so often. Rats are fed on a variety of grains, hemp and sunflower seeds, dried bread, cooked potatoes, and carrots. This food must be offered in a bowl inside the cage; it gets dirty quickly and the animals drag it around. Therefore, about twice the food amounts are needed, and during the daily feeding all leftovers must be painstakingly removed.

Since only optimally fed food animals are in excellent health and prolific—and only top-quality feeders are good enough for our animals—everything points towards recommending the commercial diet. Note that this food will spoiled if stored improperly. The food should be stored in a cool, dry, and well-ventilated location so that no mold can develop.

Breeding Conditions:

Light: Mice and rats preferred subdued light; constantly dark rooms are unsuitable. Albinos are especially sensitive to sunlight. It does not matter whether they receive natural or artificial light.

Temperatures: The best temperature is 19-23°C. If the animals are kept cool all the time or exposed to constant changes in temperature, they catch cold easily, which, if not recognized and treated promptly, will often kill them. Drafts must also be avoided.

Humidity: Mice are most comfortable at medium relative air humidity; the optimum is around 40-60%, for rats the lower, for mice the upper value applies.

They must always have drinking water available. If pellets are fed, the animals die if they are left without water for 1-2 days since the dry food is a dehydrator. The thirsty animals will attack their weaker cage mates and eat them. It is important to use good quality drinking water. Tap water with little chlorination that is also suitable for human consumption is the cheapest and easiest way to satisfy the needs of the rodents.

Notes:

Small-scale breeding:

Mice: To breed mice a group of 1 male with 2-5 females has proven ideal. If several males are kept together, they will fight until they have established a pecking order. The males will constantly bite each other's testicles, tails, and hind feet. Nursing females are unnecessarily bothered by the presence of several males. On the other hand, the time when a female that has just given birth can mate again is so short, that pregnant females should not be kept separate. If only a few mice are needed and it suffices if the female has a litter every 6-7 weeks, separation is recommended. A female is fertile again only 5-24 hours after giving birth. If she does not mate during that period, she will not be receptive again until 2-4 days after weaning her young, which is about 3 weeks later. Mice that do not mate regularly are fertile for about 12 hours during every 3-6 day fertility cycle. The rest period between cycles is 2-3 days for young animals and gets longer for older ones. Since animals from different breeding stock with an unfamiliar smell can get into fights, it is best to start a breeding group by placing all the animals into a clean cage that is free of smells at the same time. Animals from the same cage share the same nest odor and are used to each other. Otherwise, the animals should be observed for a few days to make sure the get along. Newly weaned mice are best for starting a new breeding setup: but they should be kept separated by gender for another 4-5 weeks.

When females give birth for the first time, they will often eat their litter. Later this should not happen anymore if they are in a setup where they are not often disturbed. If a mouse dies in a group, a new female can usually be introduced without problems. To introduce a new male, however, it is best to move all the animals to a cage that is free of mouse odors.

Since mice have litters regularly, you can calculate how many you need and how many breeders are required for a steady supply. This determines the number of cages. At least two containers must be available for weaned young, one for males, one for females, since these should not breed. If adult mice are used as feeders, the males should be used first. If the setup has been running for a while, old animals can be culled once a new breeding group has been established. Lastly, the young females are used as food. It helps to keep notes of when the groups have been established and when litters are produced. This helps keep determine when the young must be separated from their parents and when the breeders should be replaced.

Mouse urine smells awful so that breeding mice in human living spaces is only recommended for those with insensitive noses. If kept clean, a limited number of mice can be bred in an apartment without scaring away visitors. If no suitable spare room is available, as for example a basement or a green house, the biggest problem is where to put the cages. We like the solution of one vivarium enthusiast in Berlin: The containers are stored on shelves in the bathroom, which has the advantage of being close to water. However, the sinks and the bathtub must be disinfected before people use them. Frequent cleaning of the cages, every 3-5 days depending on population density, is necessary when keeping the cages in an apartment, and it is recommended anyway. If a spare set of cages is kept ready, cleaning is a lot easier: all the extras are filled with 2-4 cm of fresh substreate. The animals are moved to the clean cages and the lids closed immediately. The dirty cages can then be cleaned thoroughly. Mice are best grasped by the root of their tail. With some experience, grabbing them by the lose skin around the neck is also possible; hold just tightly enough that the skin is taught. If they are pinched too hard, they can be injured.

Rats: For rats a gender ratio of 1:2-3 has proven ideal. Such a breeding group is housed in a 60 x 35 cm cage and stays together at all times. If all the females have litters at the same time, it is better to remove some of the young and use them as food before they are weaned. The remaining young grow up stronger and have more space.

Rats are more aggressive towards rats that smell differently than mice are; therefore, the animals must be introduced to each other in an odor-free cage. For the rest of the time rats get along peacefully, even the males. Cleanliness of the cages is the first law, just as for mice, in the interest of both the animals as well as the keepers. To move them, rats are grasped with one hand by the root of their tail, which often causes them to defecate. Calm movements will keep the animals from biting. Be careful when trying to recapture an escaped rat. Gloves will protect your hands from being bitten by the excited animal.

Breeding rats requires a lot of space because of the size of the animals, and most likely it is not practical to try in an apartment. Except for the smallest setups, a separate room is recommended.

Large-scale breeding:

Mice: For large-scale breeding a gender ratio of 1:4 is practical and controllable. However, the number of cages is significantly larger. Good results have been seen with 2 males and 12-15 females in cages of 60 x 35 cm.

Rats: For large-scale breeding the animals are housed at a 1-2:10 ratio in 60 x 35 cm cages. The final number of rats in the cage will be smaller as, unlike for small-scale breeding, gravid females are kept separately in nesting cages and are only returned to the breeding cage after they have weaned their young.

It is a certain disadvantage that the females have litters only every 6 weeks. However, the size of the litters and that they are usually raised flawlessly make up for this. Well-kept and well-fed rats from good stock are excellent mothers that will at most eat only their first litter.

General notes on large-scale breeding: All the information for small-scale efforts is applicable here, too. However, it is now impossible to get by without a dedicated room. It should be kept at an even temperature and ventilated without drafts. Flies should be kept out as they can transmit the dreaded salmonella. Cages are efficiently stored in racks that are set off from the wall by about 5-10 cm for better air circulation. For Makrolon tubs, movable racks of var-ious sizes are available. For rats, one might consider using wire cages for all animals except the pregnant and nursing females.

A corner with running water and a large sink for cage cleaning is indispensable; who wants to carry 30, 50, or more cages across the house to the bathroom? A strong table is also needed, preferably with a metal top that can be easily cleaned which, is used for many chores such as weighing, cage transfers, examinations, and treatments. A hose with a spray nozzle attached to the faucet is very useful. It is used to fill the water bottles so that not every bottle must be filled from the tap separately. More important than for small-scale setups is a second set of cages, so that cleaning can be done efficiently.

The larger the breeding effort, the greater the need for a quarantine room, because the risk of losing the whole stock from disease increases.

Pests and Diseases: Mice are unfortunately more susceptible than rats and require a very clean and healthy environment. To thrive both species need food of the highest quality and clean and regularly disinfected cages and water bottles. If these prerequisites are met, and the best possible breeding stock has been obtained, diseases should be rare. If new animals are acquired, they should be kept in quarantine for 4 weeks, observed carefully, and treated if necessary and possible.

Diseases that are caused by dietary mistakes have such varied symptoms that it is beyond the scope of this book to discuss them all. They can mostly be avoided by offering the animals high-quality foods (see section on Food). Of other illnesses, only the most common are mentioned here.

Parasites: The protozoans, which can infect all internal organs, must be mentioned first. Many are a natural part of the intestinal flora, as for example *Entamoeba muris* and *Lamblia muris*; they only endanger malnourished and poorly kept mice and rats. If the infection is serious, *L. muris* causes slimy feces and diarrhea. Untreated, the disease is fatal in 1-8 days but it can be cured with Metronidazol; however, it is better to kill affected animals.

Among sporozoans of the order Coccidida *Eimeria falciformis* and other species cause the so-called Coccidiosis, a disease that damages the internal organs and ultimately kills. Treatment with Sulfonamides is possible, for example Durenat (oral) or other medications that some companies have developed specifically as for example sulfaquinoxalin, sulfamethazine, sulfadimethoxin, or ormetoprim. Medications based on amprolium are also effective as well as a variety of combinations. Another Coccidida member, *Toxoplasma gondii* causes toxoplasmosis, a disease that was thought to be transmitted to humans from dogs and rodents. This can only happen, however, if the human ate raw mice and other animals. The primary source of infection is probably raw pork, beef, and other raw meat.

In mice that are bred for laboratory and food use toxoplasmosis is almost insignificant as the rodents could only get infected if they ate infected cat feces. Then, however, the disease would be fatal within a few days. If the mice are cannibalistic, the disease can be passed on.

Toxoplasma gondii uses a two-host cycle: the nonsexual reproduction can take place in a variety of hosts, all vertebrates, while the sexual reproduction only takes place in house cats and other cat-like predators. Species of the genus *Sarcocystis* also go through a two-host cycle. An interesting cycle can be observed between reticulated pythons (*Python reticulatus*) and rats (*Rattus norvegicus*). Newly imported pythons are usually infested, which suggests a wide range for these parasites. Brehm and Frank (1980) showed that the oocytes that are excreted in the snake feces are immediately infectious to rats. If the rats and reptiles are not kept clean, the oocytes are easily transmitted to the rat food by flies, cockroaches, or ants. Just a few oocytes can lead to infection. If infected by as few as 50-150 oocytes the rats will get sick with high fever, bleeding in the intestines, and often they will die. This example illustrates the importance of good hygiene!

Parasitic worms mostly infect various sections of the intestine but also the lungs, liver, and muscles. They can be discovered through fecal examinations. The most important nematodes develop directly; that is, without an intermediary host. *Syphacia* and *Aspiculuris* species grow to only a few millimeters in mice and rats. Treatment is rarely necessary; all affected animals are used as feeders and a new breeding group is started with clean stock. Mice can be an intermediary host for snake ascarid worms. *Ophidascaris* species, for example, develop in mice if infected feces from snake litter come into contact with the substrate or food of the mice. If such mice are fed to other snakes, the ascarid worm infection will spread.

The tapeworm (Class Cestodes) *Hymenol-*

epis nana reaches a length of up to 55 mm and causes inflammation of the small intestine, which can kill the mice if the infestation is strong. This tapeworm can develop directly or through an intermediary host. Several insects as for example flour beetles, beetles of the genus Dermestidae, lesser mealworm beetles, and probably flies are all potential intermediary hosts. *Hymenoleps diminuta*, which occurs primarily in rats, always uses insects as intermediary hosts. Droncit (dosage: 5 mg/kg animal) is effective against tape worms, Panacur (dosage: 10-30 mg/kg animal) or Rintal (dosage: 10-30 mg/kg animal) against nematodes.

Of insect pests, the fleas (Order Aphaniptera) are easiest to control since their non-parasitic larvae cannot develop in the substrate if it is replaced twice a week. Two species in particular dine on mice: *Leptopsylla segnis* and *Nosopsyllus fascinatus*. Rats can be infested by 57 different species of fleas; suffice to mention *Nosopsyllus fascinatus*, *Leptopsylla segnis*, and *Ctenophthalmus agyrtes*.

Of more significance are lice (Order Anoplura). Since they go through incomplete metamorphosis, spend all their development time on the same host, and suck blood during all of them; this causes significant blood loss in the host. In addition, the rodents are constantly restless if they have many lice. The lice that infest mice and rats belong to the genus *Polyplax*. Insecticides are effective at controlling infestation. The use of natural Pyrethrum preparations is recommended, as they are less toxic than synthetic poisons. Adult fleas can easily be killed with insecticides. The substrate must be destroyed, otherwise

new fleas will hatch within a few days from the pupae.

Mites (Class Acari) belong to the spider-like animals. Nymphs and adults have 4 pairs of legs (the larvae only have 6 extremities). Most mites are small, about 0.15-0.5 mm long. They can only be seen with a strong magnifying glass, or if there are so many that they can be seen as a wobbling mass.

The mites eat on or inside the skin and fur. The most important ones in mice are: *Myocoptes musculinus* and *Myobia musculi*; and in rats: *Myobia ratti*. In addition, *Demodex* and *Notoedres* species can be found. *Notoedres* and *Sarcoptes* species cause scabs on the skin of mice and rats. The skin will look crusty. According to Schmidt (1979), the following treatment is effective for mice: All affected skin areas are sprayed three times at intervals of 5 days with undiluted Euphagol-VA solution or 2% Alkylphosphate solution. Rats are bathed in a solution of Hexachlorcyclohexan. All other mites can be faught using Neguvon, or even better, Alugan powder or Antorgan solution.

Animals that have been treated with acaricides or insecticides must not be used as food for at least 14 days! Neguvon, for example, can cause paralysis in some reptiles.

Viral and bacterial diseases: Many of these diseases present with symptoms that are difficult to interpret by the lay person. Their exact identification is only possible in a laboratory setting, for example, by a veterinarian.

Thus, only the most important ones are mentioned here. Mousepox (Ectromelia) is a viral infection that can lead to high losses since it is very contagious. It is vital to use breeding stock that is free of mousepox. Infected mice make a telltale sound with their teeth; if enough animals are in the room, it can be clearly heard if they are infected.

A dreaded bacterial infection is salmonellosis, which can be caused by many species of the genus *Salmonella*, for example *Salmonella typhimurium*. Several forms of this disease are known. The chronic form is the most pernicious since sick animals infect their cage mates without appearing to be ill. The acute form expresses itself in mice with diarrhea and general weakness; after 2-4 days they die. In rats, weight loss and brown-glittering eyes and brown scabs on the skin and around the nostrils, as well as pale ears can be seen. Seventy persent of sick rats die within 1-2 weeks. There are several variations that fall in between acute and chronic and that show different symptoms. Sick animals must be killed and burnt. As a preventive measure, only highest-quality food must be purchased and stored in such a way that wild rodents cannot access it. All the animals should be protected from contact with wild rodents.

Feeding: Mice and rats are fed to strong, healthy vivarium animals, preferably alive and at their preferred feeding time. A hungry animal will attack and eat the prey quickly. You must observe the feedings to make sure every animal gets enough and interfere when quarrels arise. After 1-2 hours uneaten feeders must be removed. Adult feeders should never be left in a terrarium overnight, as they can attack and chew on vivarium animals, especially on snakes, and injure them seriously. Sometimes killing a rodent will be unavoidable. The quickest way to kill a mouse is by grabbing it by the tail and hitting it hard on the edge of a table. Alternatively, for both types of rodents, they can be grasped firmly by the head and rear from above and pulled apart with a strong motion. Not everybody can stomach this, even though these are the most painless methods for the animals. If you can or will not kill them by hand, you can suffocate them with CO_2. The CO_2 gas is pumped from a tank into a small, tightly closed until the rodent is dead.

Mice and rats are the main source of food for many small to large snakes; many snakes feed exclusively on rodents. Mice and rats are also essential for feeding large lizards like monitor lizards and tegus, small and medium crocodiles, and large frogs. Mice can also be fed to medium-sized lizards, chameleons, skinks, agamas, large water turtles, and some tortoises. Nestling mice ("pinkies") are no bigger than a large cricket or locust. They make a good food for pregnant females because of their calcium content.

Large bird spiders, scorpions, and centipedes cannot be fed on insects alone; their staple food can include pinky mice. To satisfy the protein needs of small monkeys, pinkies can also be used.

Advantages and Disadvantages:

Advantages:
- Excellent food source with many uses
- Easy to care for if prepared foods are used
- Almost noiseless except for the quiet whistling of nestlings

Disadvantages:
- Odor is unavoidable
- Requires frequent cleanings
- Takes up a lot of space

Sources

Breeding Stock

Specific information on how to acquire stock is not provided as the information goes out of date too quickly. The best sources are other hobbyists and vivarium clubs. In addition, many zoological institutions and schools might have animals available. Few zoos are willing or able to part with their breeding stock. Searching specialty magazines and the Internet can yield breeders that will provide breeding stock for a variety of food animals.

Equipment can be obtained from laboratory suppliers, breeders, and pet stores. Cultivation media can be purchased from suppliers, breeders, and pet stores.

For all supplies the Internet and a variety of specialist and professional magazines provide useful listings.

One source of scientific supplies for teachers and schools that also sells to the public and that has been around for many years is the Carolina Biological Supply Company. Their Internet address is http://www.carolina.com/, their phone number is (800) 334-5551. In addition to cages, laboratory supplies, cultivation media, and foods, they also carry a wide variety of live animals, including but not limited to: waxworms, brine shrimp, houseflies, skilkworms, freshwater and marine algae, daphnia, cockroaches, beetles, and more.

References

Books about Breeding Food Animals

Geyer, H.: Praktische Futterkunde. Alfred Kernen Verlag, Stuttgart 1957, 6. Aufl.

Jahn, J.: Lebendfutter. Lehrmeister-Bücherei Nr. 17; Albrecht Philler Verlag, Minden 1978, 2. Aufl.

Jocher, W.: Futter für Vivarientiere. Franckh'sche Verlagshandlung, Stuttgart 1975.

Kleinsteuber, E. und G. Fiedler: Futter für Terrarientiere. Neumann-Verlag, Leipzig-Radebeul, 1982.

Krumbiegel, I.: Gefangene Tiere richtig füttern. DLG-Verlagsgesellschaft, Frankfurt/Main 1976, 4. Aufl.

Webb, A. and F.: Breeding Live Food For Reptiles and Tarantulas. Fitzgerald Publishing, London, 1987.

Wyninger, R.: Insektenzucht. Verlag Eugen Ulmer, Stuttgart 1974.

Zimmermann, H.: Futtertiere von A–Z. Aquärien- und Terrarientiere – richtig ernährt. Franckh'sche Verlagsbandlung, Stuttgart, 1982.

Books for Vivarium Enthusiasts That Mention Breeding Food Animals

Aleven, J. M.: Alles über das Terrarium. Alfred Kernen Verlag, Stuttgart 1970.

Austin, O. L.: Singvögel der Welt. Rheingauer Verlagsgesellschaft, Eltville am Rhein 1976, 3. Aufl.

Berndt, T.: Kleine Terrarienkunde. Falken-Verlag, Erich Sicker, Wiesbaden 1966.

Bielfeld, H.: Prachtfinken. Verlag Eugen Ulmer, Stuttgart 1973.

Frey, H.: Das Aquarium von A bis Z. Verlag J. Neumann-Neudamm, Radebeul 1966, 7. Aufl.

Kahl, B., Gaupp, P. und Schmidt, G.: Das Terrarium. Falken-Verlag, Niedernhausen 1980.

Klingelhöffer, W. und Scherpner, C.: Terrarienkunde. Bd. 1 (Allgemeines und Technik). Alfred Kernen Verlag, Stuttgart 1955.

Klös, H.-G. und J. Lange: Tierwelt hinter Glas. Das Zoo-Aquarium Berlin. arani Verlag und Verlag Haude & Spener, Berlin, 1988.

Lilge, D. und Meeuwen, H. v.: Grundlagen der Terrarienhaltung. Landbuchverlag, Hannover 1979.

Mayland, H. J.: Das Aquarium. Falken Verlag, Niedernhausen 1975.

Mayland, H. J.: Das Süßwasser-Aquarium. Falken-Verlag, Niedernhausen 1978, 2. Aufl.

Meaden, F.: A Manual of European Bird Keeping. Blanford Press, Poole and Dorset, 1979.

Neunzig, K.: Praxis der Vogelpflege und -Züchtung (Handbuch III). Creutzsche Verlagsbuchhandlung, Magdeburg 1927.

Nietzke, G.: Die Terrarientiere, Bd. I. Verlag Eugen Ulmer, Stuttgart 1977, 2. Aufl.

Obst, F. J., K. Richter und U. Jacob: Lexikon der Terraristik. Edition Leipzig, 1984.

Ostermöler, W.: Die Aquarienfibel. Franckh'sche Verlagshandlung, Stuttgart 1976, 5. Aufl.

Paysan, K.: Beispielhafte Aquarien. Tetra-Werke, Melle 1 1978.

Redaktion Aquarienmagazin: Kosmos-Handbuch Aquarienkunde. Das Süßwasseraquarium. Franckh'sche Verlagshandlung, Stuttgart 1978.

Rimpp, K.: Das Terrarium. Ulmer Taschenbuch 27, Verlag Eugen Ulmer, Stuttgart, 1986.

Robiller, F.: Prachtfinken. Verlag J. Neumann-Neudamm, Melsungen 1978.

Sachs, W. B.: Vogel-Pflege – leicht gemacht. Franckh'sche Verlagshandlung, Stuttgart 1954.

Sachs, W. B.: Aquarienpflege leicht gemacht. Franckh'sche Verlagshandlung, Stuttgart 1977.

Schmidt, G.: Kleinsäuger. Verlag Eugen Ulmer, Stuttgart 1973.

Schulte, R.: Frösche und Kröten. Verlag Eugen Ulmer, Stuttgart 1980.

Stettler, P. H.: Handbuch der Terrarienkunde. Franckh'sche Verlagshandlung, Stuttgart 1979.

Vogel, Z.: Wunderwelt Terrarium. Verlag J. Neumann-Neudamm, Melsungen 1962.

Vogt, D. und Wermuth, H.: Knaurs Aquarien- und Terrarienbuch. Droemer Knaur, München, Zürich 1977, 2. Aufl.

Zimmermann, E.: Das Züchten von Terrarientieren. Pflege, Verhalten, Fortpflanzung. Franckh'sche Verlagshandlung, Stuttgart, 1983.

Zimmermann, H.: Tropische Frösche. Franckh'sche Verlagshandlung, Stuttgart 1979.

Specialized References on Breeding Food Animals

Vivarienkundliche Zeitschriften

(und ihre Abkürzungen, die im Literaturverzeichnis verwendet werden)

Aqu.-Mag.: Aquarien-Magazin. Monatshefte für Aquarien- und Vivarienkunde. Kosmos-Verlag, Stuttgart (bis 3/1988, danach vereint mit DATZ).

Aqu. Terr.: Aquarien Terrarien. Monatsschrift für Vivarienkunde und Zierfischzucht. Urania-Verlag, Leipzig (bis 1990, danach vereint mit DATZ).

Aquariumwereld: Monatsschrift. Offizielles Organ des „Belgische Bond voor Aquarium- en Terrariumkunde V.Z.W." (B.B.A.T.).

Aquaterra: Monatsschrift für Aquaristik und Terraristik sowie für Pflanzen- und Tierpflege im Heim. Biberist, Schweiz. (bis 1973).

AZN: AZ-Nachrichten. Mitteilungsblatt der Vereinigung for Artenschutz, Vogelhaltung und Vogelzucht (AZ) e.V. Geschäftsstelle Backnang.

Das Aquarium. Magazin für zeitgemäße Vivaristik. Birgit Schmettkamp Verlag, Bornheim 3.

DATZ: Die Aquarien- und Terrarienzeitschrift, vereinigt mit Aquarien Terrarien und aquarien magazin. Verlag Eugen Ulmer Stuttgart.

Ent. Nachr. Ber.: Entomologische Nachrichten und Berichte. Vierteljahreshefte, herausgegeben von der Entomofaunistischen Gesellschaft e.V., Leipzig.

Gef. Welt.: Gefiederte Welt. Fachzeitschrift für Vogelfreunde, Vogelpfleger und Züchter. Verlag E. Ulmer Stuttgart.

herpetofauna: Die Zeitschrift für den Terrarianer. herpetofauna-Verlags-GmbH, Weinstadt.

Lacerta: Zweimonatsblatt der Niederländischen Vereinigung für Herpetologie und Terrarienkunde.

Mittbi. Salam.: Salamandra. Zeitschrift für Herpetologie und Terrarienkunde. Herausgegeben von der Deutschen Gesellschaft für Herpetologie und Terrarienkunde e. V., Frankfurt am Main.

Sauria: Die Zeitschrift der Terrarianer. Herausgegeben von der Terrariengemeinschaft Berlin e.V.

Terra: Zeitschrift der Beigischen Vereinigung für Terrarienkunde und Herpetologie, Merksem.

Trochilus: Eine Fachzeitschrift über tropische Vögel. Ab 1991: Tropische Vögel. Vierteljahresschrift. Herausgegeben von Dr. Karl-L. Schuchmann, Bonn.

Wochenschr.: Wochenschrift für Aquarien- und Terrarienkunde. Verlag Gustav Wenzel und Sohn, Braunschweig (ab 1951 mit DATZ vereinigt).

Arnold, A.: Erfahrungen bei der Haltung der afrikanischen Höhlengrille Pholeogryllus geertsi Chopard (Saltatoria). Ent. Nachr. Ber. **27** (5), 230–231, 1983.

Badeda, S.: Fliegenmaden als Aufzuchtfutter. Gef. Welt **111** (4), 109, 1987.

Ballasina, D. L. P.: Ervaringen met de treksprinkhaan Locusta migratoria migratorioides. Lacerta **40** (6), 102–107, 1982.

Bartholdi, P.: Einfache Zucht der Heimchen (Hausgrille). Mittbl. Salam. **3**, 51–52, 1962.

Bartholdi, P.: Stubenfliegenzucht – ohne Geruchsbildung. Aquaterra **3**, 22–24 (1 Abb.), 1966.

Bauer: Frisches Lebendfutter für unsere Exoten. Drosophila. AZN, 248–249, 1975.

Baumgartner, E.: Meine Heimchenzucht. Gef. Welt **105** (12), 244, 1981.

Berndt, K.-P.: Calliphoriden-Zucht ohne Geruchsbelästigung. Angew. Parasitol. **10,** 233–236, 1969.

Bertram, G.: Die Zucht von Enchyträen. Wertvoll – aber nicht immer. Das Aquarium **1** (1), 6–7, (1 Abb.), 1967.

Biesôt, T.: Het kweken van springstaarten (Collembola). Lacerta **47** (2), 61–62, 1988/89.

Bitsch, H.: Ein leckeres Zubrot für Aquarienfische: Wachsmotten. Aqu.-Mag. **14** (4), 160–161, (2 Abb.), 1980.

Böhm, O.: Die indische Stabheuschrecke als Terrarienpflegling und Futterquelle. DATZ **29** (7), 244–245 (3 Abb.), 1976.

Brandt, A.: Warum keine Winterzucht der Schmeißfliege? Gef. Welt **88,** 97–98, 1964.

Claassen, L.: Voedsel problemen? Het vangen van insecten en her kweken van vliegen. Lacerta **19** (1), 3 u. 7–8, 1960.

Cock, J. J.: Het voederen met larven van de wasmot. Lacerta **10** (8), 60–61, 1952.

Dahlke, H.: Zucht von Artemia salina. Aqu. Terr. **3** (3), 91–92, 1956.

Daiss, S.: Gryllus domesticus als Futtertiere. herpetofauna **1** (3), 16–17, 1979.

De Batist, P.: De reuzenmeelworm. Aquariumwereld **37** (2), 44-46 (2 Abb.), 1984.

De Batist, P.: Nogmaals de reuzenmeelworm. Aquariumwereld **38** (4), 96, 1985.

De Batist, P.: Problemlose Fliegenzucht. DATZ **44** (5), 318–321, 1991.

De Batist, P.: Voedseldieren: Tenebrio molitor. Terra **27** (7), 95, 1991.

De Batist, P. en Van Maele, A.: Voedseldieren: Galleria mellonella. Terra **25** (8),
138, 1989.

De Batist, P. en Van Tomme, G.: Kweeken
met de vleugelloze Afrikaanse vlieg.
Aquariumwereld **38** (5), 114–116, 1985.

Dittmar, H.: Daphnia-Zucht in kleinen
Behältern. Das Aquarium **1** (3), 34–35,
1967.

Dobroruka, L. J.: Pholeogryllus geertsi
CHOPARD 1923, eine afrikanische Höhlengrille. Aqu. Terr. **19** (8), 278–279
(2 Abb.), 1972.

Dohse, H.: Artemia en gros. Ein Beitrag
zur Aufzucht und Vermehrung von Artemia salina. DATZ **23** (11), 348–350
(1 Abb.), 1970.

Dohse, H.: Das Artemium. Die kleine
Lebendfutterfabrik. I. DATZ **24** (12),
413–415 (2 Abb.), 1971 – II. DATZ **25**
(1), 34–36 (1 Abb.), 1972. – III. DATZ
25 (2), 61–63 (2 Abb.), 1972.

Dohse, H.: Artemien automatisch. DATZ
26 (2), 68–70 (3 Abb.), 1973.

Dohse, H.: Artemia-Zystenenthüllung.
DATZ **31** (9), 320–323 (8 Abb.), 1978.

Dürr, K. L.: Die Anlage von Protozoen-
reinkulturen. Wochenschr. **44** (3), 88–91
(4 Abb.), 1950.

Eberlé, W.: Haltung und Zucht von Enchyträen. Aquarium **3** (5), 54–55, 1948.

Eck, F. en G. van: Een kweek van regen-
wormen. Lacerta **49** (3), 95–96, 1991.

Eckert, G.: Zucht von Grindal-Würmchen.
DATZ **12** (5), 156–157, 1959.

Ehlert, B. W.: Die Mediterrane Zweifleck-
grille Gryllus bimaculatus de Greer
(Orthoptera, Gryllidae) – ein hochwerti-
ges Futterinsekt. Teile 1–3. Sauria **4** (1),
11–17, (2), 25–33, (3), 29–34, 1982.

Emmert, U.: Drosophila melanogaster, ein
vergessenes Fischfutter. DATZ 7 (1),
13–14 (3 Abb.), 1954.

Essmann, U.: Ertragreiche Zucht des Getreideschimmelkäfers (Alphitobius ovatus). DATZ **29** (3), 105–107 (1 Abb.),
1976.

Essmann, U.: Der gute Tip: Die Zucht von
„Essigälchen" ohne Geruchsbelästigung.
Das Aquarium **20** (H. 200), 79, 1986.

Eysden, E. van: Wasmotten, Sprinkhanen
en Kakkerlakken. Lacerta **21** (1), 4–5,
1962.

Fischer, H.: Kleinstfutter kein Problem.
Wochenschr. **44** (4), 120–122 (1 Abb.),
1950.

Fischer, H.: Kleinstfischfutter. DATZ **4**
(4), 99–101 (1 Abb.), 1951.

Florschütz, P. A.: Nog iets over de kweek
van fruitvliegen. Lacerta **15** (5), 47, 1957.

Friederich, U.: Das Züchten von Futter-
insekten. Voliere 7 (6), 232–237, 1984.

Friedrich, H.: Grindalzucht – salonfähig
gemacht. Aqu. -Mag. **1** (7), 298, 1967.

Fritz, H.: Fischfutter aus dem „Bienenkorb"
(die Zucht von Taufliegenmaden). Aqu.-
Mag. **1** (10), 420–422 (4 Abb.), 1967.

Fuchs K.: Insektenzuchten und deren Verwendung im Zoo Innsbruck. Gef. Welt
104 (7), 132–134, 1980.

Geus, A.: Über ein Massenauftreten von
Mycetaea hirta MARSH. (Coleoptera)
in Kulturen von Enchytraeus albidus.
DATZ **14** (4), 122, 1961.

Geyer, H. und Becker, R.: Das „Grindal"-
Würmchen. DATZ **5** (7), 183–184, 1952.

Geyer, H.: Zusätzliches zu dem Kapitel
„Grindal"-Würmchen = Enchytraeus
buchholzi (VEJDOVSKYV). DATZ **6** (4),
97, 1953.

Gibson, L.: Some sources of live food. Avi-
cult. Mag. **86** (1), 33–39, 1980.

Goger, R.: Schimmelkäferzucht. Get. Welt **108** (5), 144, 1984.

Goger, R.: Zucht der Essigfliege als Futter fiir Vögel und Fische. Gef. Welt **108** (5), 145, 1984.

Greve, W.: Brachionus plicatilis–ein Rädertier eröffnet neue Wege in der Meeresaquaristik. DATZ **28** (11), 394–395 (1 Abb.), 1975.

Grindal, N.: Ein anderer Enchyträus, Enchytraeus buchholzi, und die Geschichte seiner Entdeckung als Futtertier für unsere Aquarienfische. DATZ **9** (2), 44–46, 1956.

Hagedoorn, F. H. J.: Een behuizing voor de krekelkweek. Lacerta **44** (10/11), 186–187, 1986.

Hagedoorn, F.: De kweek van de grote wasmot (Gaileria mellonella). Lacerta **47** (3), 81–84, 1989.

Hausberger, A.: Heimchenzucht. Gef. Welt **81,** 55–56 (3 Abb.), 1957.

Heeland, R.: Grundschule der Aquaristik. Fischzucht ist auch Futterzucht. Das Aquarium **15** (H. 147), 450–456, 1981.

Helbig, W.: Getreideschimmelkäferlarven als Futtertiere. Gef. Welt **109** (10), 280, 1985.

Held, B.: Meine Grillenzucht. Gef. Welt **83,** 217–218, 1959.

Hesse, U.: Rädertierchenkultur als Aufzuchtfutter. [Süßwasser]. DATZ **17** (9), 282–283, 1964.

Hoppe, R.: Heuschrecken als Weichfresserfutter. Gef. Welt **87,** 34–35, 1963.

Hoppe, R.: Über die Zucht von Lebendfutter (Grillen, Heimchen, Käfer, Asseln). Gef. Welt **89,** 171–172, 1965.

Hoppe, R. und Hoppe M.: Die Wachsmotte als ideales Lebendfutter. Gef. Welt **87,** 77, 1963.

Horn, H. und Horn, W.: Über die Zucht von Wasserflöhen. Aqu. Terr. **23** (8), 270–274 (3 A bb.), 1976.

Horn, H. und Horn, W.: Noch einmal über die Zucht von Wasserflöhen. Aqu. Terr. **23** (10), 345 (1 Abb.), 1976.

Horn, K.: Mikrozucht im Einkochtopf. Aqu.-Mag. **18** (8), 374, 1984.

Horrer, F.: Zucht von Ägyptischen Wanderheuschrecken Locusta migratoria. Gef. Welt **113** (6), 177–178, 1989.

Horst, J. Th. ter: Wandelende takken. Lacerta **18** (2), 9–11, 1959.

Irtz, P.: Heimchen als Futtertiere. DATZ **13** (10), 318–319, 1960.

Jaenen, A.: Een goed georganiseerde krekelkweek. Aquariumwereld **44** (12), 269–271, 1991.

Janssen, H. A.: Een andere manier om fruitvliegen te voeren aan jonge salamanders. Lacerta **44** (10/11), 193, 1986.

Kießling, G.: Pantoffeltierchenzucht. Aqu. Terr. **1** (4/5), 78–79, 1954.

Kirschke, S.: Meine Mehlwurmzucht. l.–3. Teil. Gef. Welt **109** (4), 104–106, (5), 128–130, (6), 161, 1985.

Kirschke, S.: Hausgrillenzucht. Gef. Welt **114** (5), 154–155, 1990.

Klein, H.: Einrichtung einer Mehlwurmgroßzucht. Gef. Welt **83,** 97–98, 1959.

Klöss, J.: Heimchenzucht leicht gemacht. Gef. Welt **82,** 73–74, 1958.

Knaack, J.: „Mikro"-Älchen - Die Gattung Turbatrix. Aqu. Terr. **5** (1), 21–24, 1958.

Kofahl, U.: Taufliegenzucht: Ausbruchsicher - geruchlos - ergiebig. Aqu.-Mag. **21** (7), 292–294, 1987.

Körber, U.: Futter für Wanderheuschrecken. Aqu. -Mag. **18** (5), 249, 1984.

Körber, U.: Zusatz von Torf bei der Obstfliegenzucht. Aqu.-Mag. **18** (7), 351, 1984.

Körber, U.: „Die achte Plage: Heuschrekken". Aqu.-Mag. **20** (3), 126–129, 1986.

Kracht, W.: Mehlwurmzucht. Gef. Welt **83,** 137–138, 1959.

Kracht, W.: Betrachtungen über das Lebendfutter. Gef. Welt **85,** 76–78, 1961.

Kremlitschka, O.: Mehlwürmerzucht. Gef. Welt **83,** 56–57, 1959.

Kremlitschka, O.: Der Getreideschimmelkäfer. Gef. Welt **89,** 117–118, 1965.

Kroon, V. A.: Een vliegensluis. Lacerta **41** (5)185–87, 1983.

Kuijten, P.: Gouden torren: het is niet alles goud, wat er blinkt. [Rosenkäfer]. Lacerta **41** (7), 129–131, 1983.

Lange, J. und R. Kaiser: Ohne Plankton geht es nicht. Probleme bei der Zucht von Korallenfischen. TI internat. Sd. Nr. **92,** 3 S., 1989.

Lanting, J.: Over de kweek van huiskrekels. Lacerta **23** (12), 99, 1965.

Laurens, B.: Enige opmerkingen over voederdieren en de kweek van de huiskrekel (Acheta domestics). Lacerta **47** (1), 15–18, 1988.

Laurens, B.: De kweek van treksprinkhanen. Lacerta **47** (4), 122–125, 1989.

Legro, Ir. R. A. H.: Drosophila als voedseldier. Lacerta **15** (5), 33–36, 1957.

Leistner, F.: Enchyträenzucht. Aqu. Terr. **1** (4/5), 91–92, 1954.

Ley, J.: Wasserflöhe aus dem Eimer. DATZ **44** (2), 112-113, 1991.

Maleck, W.: Betreff: „Mikro – Ein immer verfügbares, praktisches Lebendfutter", DATZ 7/88. DATZ **41** (11), 505, 1988.

Mantel, P.: Het kweken van fruitvliegen (Drosophila). Lacerta **48** (1), 25–26, 1989.

Mantel, P.: De huisvlieg (Musca domestica) als voederdier. Lacerta **47** (6), 165–167, 1989.

Marinkelle, C. J.: Een eenvoudige en hygiënische methode voor het kweken van meelwormen. Lacerta **19** (9), 71–72, 1961.

Mau, K. G.: Ein Beitrag zur Zucht der Großen Wachsmotte (Galleria mellonella). Gef. Welt **97,** 46–50 (5 Abb.), 1973.

Mau, K. G.: Ein Beitrag zur Zucht der Indischen Feldgrille (Gryllus bimaculatus) DE GREER. Gef. Welt **100,** 239–244 (9 Abb.), 1976.

Mau, K. G.: Zur Zucht der Indischen Feldgrille. DATZ **31** (10), 358–359 (2 Abb.), 1978.

Mayland, H. J.: Die siebte Plage (Heuschreckenzucht). Aqu.-Mag. **1** (12), 519–521, 1967.

Meeuwes, M. Th.: Wasmottenkweek. Lacerta **40** (7), 147, 1982.

Mehner, H.: Enchyträenzucht und Milbenvernichtung. DATZ **14** (8), 253, 1961.

Mickoleit, E.: Futtertierzucht. [Heimchen]. Mittbl. Salam. **3,** 61–62, 1962.

Milautzcki: Enchyträen – ein vorzügliches Lebendfutter. AZN, 140, 1976.

Möller, K.: Praktische Regenwurmzucht. Aqu. Terr. **1** (9/10), 190, 1954.

Moustafa, U.: Die Zucht der echten Heuschrecke als wertvolles Lebendfutter [Wanderheuschrecke]. Gef. Welt **100,** 97, 1976.

Mudrack, W.: Zucht der Sardinischen Grille. Aqu.-Mag. **4** (6)1280, 1970.

Mudrack, W.: Man muß nicht die Nase rümpfen: Die geruchlose Stubenfliegenzucht. Aqu.-Mag. **13** (12), 623–624, 1979.

Müller, W.: Die Insektenfütterung exotischer Zierfische. Aqu. Terr. **3** (3), 89–91, 1956.

Müller, W.: Grindalwurmzucht – richtig gemacht. Aqu. Terr. **5** (7), 214–215, 1958.

Müllcr-Langenbeck, G.: Die Einrichtung einer Heuschreckenzuchtanlage. DATZ **17** (3), 92–93 (3 Abb.), 1964.

Musil, A.: Mehlwürmer. Gef. Welt. **83,** 18, 1959.

Mußler, E.: Ein neues Verfahren zur problemlosen Zucht von Fruchtfliegen. Trochilus 1982 (3), 41– 42, 1982.

Nachstedt, J.: aus: Zusammenfassende Berichte über die bekannten und beliebten Aphyosemion-Arten. 6. Aphyosemion calabaricus E. Ahl,. [Grindalwurmzucht]. DATZ **5** (6), 145 –146, 1952.

Nestler, L.: Die Zucht der stummelflügligen Form der Tau- oder Obstfliege. Aqu. Terr. **7** (5), 153–154, 1960.

Oeser, R.: Massenzucht von Drosophila. DATZ **13** (6), 185–186, 1960.

Oeser, R.: Fliegenzucht. DATZ **4** (5), 134–135, 1951.

Offreins, H. W.: Het kweken van vliegen. Lacerta **16** (6-7), 46, 1958.

Paulsen, J.-P.: Zur Haltung von Futtertieren. DATZ **29** (8), 283–286 (6 Abb.), 1976.

Pavel, D.: Grindal, ein feines Ergänzungsfutter für Aquariumfische. Das Aquarium **20** (H. 207), 480, 1986.

Pederzani, H.-A.: Zucht von Daphnien – machbar oder nicht? 1: Was fressen Wasserflöhe? Aqu. Terr. **29** (1), 10–11, 1982.

Pederzani, H. -A.: Daphnienfutter – machbar oder nicht? 2: Der Fortpflanzungsmodus – die Klippe der Zucht. Aqu. Terr. **29** (2). 46–48, 1982.

Peters, K. M.: Der gezielte Einsatz von Artemia salida. Das Aquarium **17** (H. 163), 19–24, 1983.

Pohlmann, G.: Er eignet sich auch als Futter für Frösche und Fische! [Speisebohnenkäfer Acanthoscelides obtectus Say]. Mittbl. Salam. **5,** 185–186, 1964

Printz, W.: Grundschule der Aquaristik. Fischfutter aus Futterkuluturen selbst gezüchtet. Das Aquarium **19** (H. 187), 19–21, 1985.

Printz, W.: Grundschule der Aquaristik. Fischfuitter aus Futterkulturen 11. Das Aquarium **19** (H. 192). 317–320, 1985

Quitschau, K.: Beobachtungen an Artemia salina. Aqu. Terr. **14** (10), 328–333 (5 Abb., 1 Tab.), 1967.

Quitschau, K.: Landasseln als Zierfischfutter. Aqu. Terr. **23** (2), 64–65 (1 Abb.), 1976.

Reuter, K.: Ein wertvolles Futterinsekt: das Hieimchen. Gef. Welt **89,** 13–16, 1965.

Richter, K.: Hausgemachte Würmer: Enchyträen. Aqu.-Mag. **14** (5), 224–227, 1980.

Rössel, D.: Mikro. Ein immer verfügbares, praktisches Lebendfutter. DATZ **41** (7), 248–249, 1988.

Rusek, J.: Springschwänze – eine willkommene Beikost für unsere Pfleglinge. Aqu.-Mag. **5** (7), 300–303 (11 Abb.), 1971.

Sarring, G.: Larve des Getreideschimmelkäfers – zu wenig beachtet. Gef. Welt **92,** 136–137, 1968.

Sauer, H. F.: Die Fruchtfliege als Fischfutter. Aqu. Terr. **2** (5), 155-156, 1955.

Schabitz, W.: Das erste Aufzuchtfutter für unsere Jungfische. DATZ **7** (11), 291–295 (13 Abb.), 1954.

Schernekau, J.: Züchtung der Stubenfliege. Gef. Welt **98,** 31–32, 1974.

Schiller, H.: Erfahrungen mit Futterkulturen. Springschwänze – Rädertiere – Taufliegen. Aqu. Terr. **5** (5), 150–152, 1958.

Schlagentweith, K.: Ergänzende Bemerkungen zur Heimzucht von Daphnien. DATZ **31** (6), 214–215, 1978.

Schmidt, B.: Plankton für Seewasseraquarien. DATZ **31** (11), 390–391, 1978.

Schmidt, H. R. und Schmidt B.: Neu im Fachhandel: Tropisches Plankton. Aqu. Mag. **13** (4), 170–171 (2 Abb.), 1979.

Schneider, P.: Erfolgreiche Mehlwurmzucht. Get. Welt **83,** 37, 1959.

Schöne, H.: Die Zucht von Zooplankton im Seewasser. I–V. I: Aqu. Terr. **23** (5/6), 177–179 (5 Abb.), 1976. – II: **23** (7), 242–246 (10 Abb.), 1976. – III: **23** (9), 294–295 (1 Abb.), 1976. – IV: **23** (12), 418–420 (6 Abb.), 1976. – V: **24** (3), 82–85 (10 Abb.), 1977.

Schöne, H.: Asseln aus der Streubtichse. Aqu. Terr. **26** (2), 50–51 (3 Abb.), 1979.

Schöne. H.: Wir züchten Salinenkrebschen. Aqu. Terr. **27** (2), 46–48 (6 Abb.), 1980.

Schöne, H.: Über die Zucht des Rädertiers Brachionus plicatilis. Aqu. Terr. **27** (8), 264–266 (5 Abb.), 1980.

Schoenen, P.: Kleine Futterkunde. – Aquarienfische – richtig ernährt, Aqu.-Mag. **12** (12), 588–592 (4 Abb.), 1978.

Schöpfel, H.: Rationelle Zucht der Tau- oder Essigfliege. Aqu. Terr. **25** (6), 186–187 (3 Abb.), 1978.

Siepe, A.: Lebendes Standardfutter: Salinenkrebschen. (Die rationelle Zucht von Artemia salina). Aqu.-Mag. **11** (4), 154–159 (10 Abb.), 1977.

Spies, G.: Meeresplanktonzucht. Aqu.-Mag. **21** (11), 468–471, 1987.

Stark, I.: Das Heimchen - ein wertvolles Futtertier. Get. Welt **112** (12), 357, 1988.

Stark, I.: Die Zucht von Stabheuschrecken. Gef. Welt **112** (11), 322–323, 1988.

Stark, I.: Der große Mehlwurm Tenebrio obscurus. [?Zophobas morio]. Gef. Welt **113** (1), 22, 1989.

Stein, K.-H.: Eine automatische Futterversorgung mit Taufliegen, Drosophila. Aqu. Terr. **11** (4), 127–128 (3 Abb.), 1964.

Steiner, G.: Die Massenzucht des Pantoffeltierchens (Paramecium caudatum). Wochenschr. **43** (10), 284–285, 1949.

Steinigeweg, W.: Die Stabheuschrecke als Lebendfutter. Gef. Welt **100,** 12–14 (2 Abb.), 1976.

Sterzel, B.: Grindal – kann man in Massen züchten! DATZ **42** (3), 181–183, 1989.

Stettler, P. H.: De kweek van huiskrekels. Lacerta **15** (3), 19–20, 1956.

Stettler, P. H.: Südländische Grillen (Gryllus bimaculatus) als Futtertiere. Aquaterra **3,** [9–10], 1966.

Stüben, M.: Fliegenzucht mit einfachen Mitteln. Aqu.-Mag. **8** (8), 334–337 (6 Abb.), 1974.

Stute, E.: Pflege und Zucht von Springschwänzen. DATZ **42** (10), 626 627, 1989.

Stute, E.: Grindal – die Erdzuchtmethode. Mit Anerkennungen zur Beschreibung der Grindalzucht auf Schaumstoff. DATZ **43** (6), 369–370, 1990.

Stute, E.: Zucht von Fruchtfliegen. Drosophila melanogaster und D. hydei. DATZ **44** (1), 50–52, 1991.

Suttner, R.: Fruchtfliegen als Fischfutter. DATZ **43** (8), 491–492, 1990.

Tannert, R.: Die Zucht von Heimchen und amerikanischen Riesenschaben. DATZ **9** (2), 46–48 (1 Abb.), 1956.

Tomey, W. A.: Das „geschdite" Artemia-Ei. Neue Methoden zur Erbrütung und Konservierung. Aqu.-Mag. **12** (9), 448–451 (5 Abb.), 1978.

Trapp, F.: Die Aufzucht von Salinenkrebschen ist lohnend. DATZ **23** (1), 25–27 (2 Abb.), 1970.

Trempenau, H.: „Mikro"-Zucht und Verwendung. Wochenschr. **43** (4), 82–83, 1949.

Uchelen, E. van: Een zelfgebouwde vliegenval. Lacerta **45** (6), 89–94, 1987.

Van Tomme, G.: Voedseldieren: Blaptica dubia, Argentijnse boskakkerlak. Aquariumwereld **44** (11), 248, 1991.

Van Tomme, G.: Voedseldieren: Collembola. Terra **27** (8), 111, 1991.

Verein für Aquarien- und Terrarienfreunde in Varel i. O.: Die „hygienische" Enchyträenzucht. DATZ **12** (9), 285–286, 1959.

Vergoossen, P.: Eenvoudige voedingsbodem voor het kweken van fruitvliegen. Lacerta **43** (6), 118–119, 1985.

Vogel, J.: Meine Zucht des Großen Schwarzkäfers (Zophobas morio). Voliere **10** (4), 122–124, 1987.

Vogel, J.: Meine Grillen- und Heimchenzucht. Voliere **11** (4), 106–109, 1988.

Vogel, J.: Die Zucht des Getreideschimmelkäfers (Alphitobius diaperinus). Voliere **11** (5), 146–148, 1988.

Walter, H. A.: Geht's nicht auch einfacher? Bemerkungen zur Zucht von Drosophila. DATZ **20** (4), 123–124, 1967.

Weischner, M.: Der Große Schwarzkäfer als Futterinsekt. Zophobas morio. Gef. Welt **113** (3), 89, 1989.

Zahn, M.: Aufzucht von Salinenkrebschen im Aquarium Düsseldorf. DATZ **25** (9), 321-323 (1 Abb.), 1972.

Zahn, M.: Ausweg aus der Lebendfuttermisere: Der pflegeleichte Wasserfloh [Moina macrocopa]. Aqu.-Mag. **12** (11), 526–527 (5 Abb.), 1978.

Zimmermann, H.: Das Insektarium eines Aqua-Terrarianers. Aqu.-Mag. **11** (1), 12–19 (16 Abb.), 1977.

Specialized References on Breeding Food Animals not Mentioned in the Text

Esterbauer, H.: Aufzucht von Lebendfutter: Lepisma saccarina, das Silberfischchen. DATZ **26** (7), 250–251 (1 Abb.), 1973.

Klausnitzer, B.: Ein neues Futter für Terrarientiere? [Blaps mucronata]. Aqu. Terr. **20** (5), 162–164 (6 Abb.), 1973.

Leeuwen, F. R. van: De spektor als voedseldier. [Speckkäfer]. Lacerta **41** (6), 110–111, 1983.

Lieder, U. und Helms, C.: Über die Massenzucht von Chironomidenlarven. Aqu. Terr. **29** (11), 373–375, 1982.

Oeser, R.: Zufällig... [Kleiner Mistkäfer]. Mittbi. Salam. **4,** 125-126, 1963.

Veenendaal, R. L.: Een methode voor het kweeken van de rijstmot (Corcyra cephalonica). Lacerta **44** (6), 103–104, 1986.

Further Readings

Beier, M.: Phasmida (Stab- oder Gespenstheuschrecken). Handb. Zool. **4** (2) 2/10, Verlag Walter de Gruyter, Berlin 1968.

Beier, M.: Saltatoria (Heuschrecken und Grillen). Handb. Zool. **4** (2) 2/9, Verlag Walter de Gruyter, Berlin 1972.

Beier, M.: Blattariae (Schaben). Handb. Zool. **4** (2) 2/13, Verlag Walter de Gruyter, Berlin 1974.

Bergerard, J.: Etude de la parthénogénèse thélytoque facultative d'un Phasmide (Clitumnus extradentatus Br.). Proc. 10. int. Congr. Entomol. 1956, Montreal, **2**, 997–1001, 1958.

Brehm, H. und Frank, W.: Der Entwicklungskreislauf von Sarcocystis singasporensis ZAMAN und COLLEG, im End- und Zwischenwirt. Z. Parasitenk. **62,** 15 30, 1980.

Buch, W.: Der Regenwurm im Garten. Ulmer Taschenbuch 21, Veriag Eugen Ulmer, Stuttgart, 1986.

Burla, H.: Systematik, Verbreitung und Ökologie der Drosophila-Arten der Schweiz. Rev. Suisse Zool. **58** (2), 22–175 (46 Abb., 17 Tab.), 1951.

Caudell, A. N.: Pycnoscelus surinamensis LINNAEUS (Orthoptera); on Its Nymphs and the Damage it Does to Rose Bushes. Proc. ent. Soc. Wash. **27** (8), 154–157, 1925.

Chopard, L.: La Biologie des Orthoptères. Edit. Paul Lechevalier, Paris 1938.

Clark, J. T.: Stick and Leaf Insects. Verlag Barry Shurlock, Winchester 1974.

Dambach, M. und Lichtenstein, L.: Zur Ethologie der afrikanischen Grille Phaeophilacris spectrum SAUSSURE. Z. Tierpsychol. **46,** 14–29, 1978.

Dietrich, G. und Kalle, K.: Allgemeine Meereskunde. Eine Einführung in die Ozeanographie. Verlag Gebrüder Borntraeger, Berlin Nikolassee 1957.

Duda, O.: Drosophilidae. Fliegen paläarkt. Region, Bd VI 1, **58** g, Verlag E. Schweizerbart, Stuttgart 1935.

Dunger, W.: Tiere im Boden. 3. Aufl. Die Neue Brehm-Bücherei 327, A. Ziemsen Verlag, Wittenberg 1983.

Eisenbeis, G. und Wichard, W.: Atlas zur Biologie der Bodenarthropoden. Gustav Fischer Verlag, Stuttgart u. New York 1985.

Frank, W.: Parasitologie. Verlag Eugen Ulmer, Stuttgart 1976.

Freude, H., Harde, K. W. und Lohse, G. A.: Die Käfer Mitteleuropas Bd. 8. Goecke und Evers Verlag, Krefeld 1969.

Frömming, E.: Biologic der mitteleuropäischen Landgastropoden. Duncker Humblot, Berlin 1954.

Geisler, H.: Mehlwürmer und Gregarinen. Gef. Welt **87,** 137, 1963.

Geus, A.: Über das Vorkommen von Gregarinen in Insekten und deren Larven. Gef. Welt **87,** 117–118, 1963.

Gisin, H.: Collembolenfauna Europas. Mus. Hist. nat., Genève, 1960.

Godan, D.: Schadschnecken. Verlag Eugen Ulmer, Stuttgart 1979.

Gruner, H.-E.: Crustaceen V. Isopoda. Tierw. Deutschl. **53,** Verlag Gustav Fischer, Jena 1966.

Grzimeks Tierleben. Band 1: Niedere Tiere. Band II: Insekten. Deutscher Taschenbuch Verlag, München 1979.

Handschin, E.: Urinsekten oder Apterygota (Protura, Collembola, Diplura und Thysanura). Tierw. Deutschl. **16,** Verlag Gustav Fischer, Jena 1929.

Harz, K.: Die Geradflügler Mitteleuropas. Verlag Gustav Fischer, Jena 1957.

Harz, K.: Geradflügler oder Orthopteren. Tierw. Deutschl. **46,** Verlag Gustav Fischer, Jena 1960.

Haydak, M. H.: Influence of the Protein Level of the Diet on the Longevity of Cockroaches. Ann. ent. Soc. Amer. **46,** 547–560, 1953.

Hennig, W.: Diptera (Zweiflügler). Handb. Zool. **4** (2) 2/31, Verlag Walter de Gruyter, Berlin 1973.

Herford, G. M.: Observations on the Biology of Bruchus obtectus SAY, with Special Reference to the Nutritional Factors. Z. angew. Ent. **21** (1), 26–50, 1936.

Hoffmann, K.-H.: Der Einfluß der Temperatur auf die chemische Zusammensetzung von Grillen (Gryllus, Orthopt.). Oecologia **13** (2), 147–175, 1973.

Hoffmann, K.-H.: Wirkung von konstanten und tagesperiodisch alternierenden Temperaturen auf Lebensdauer, Nahrungsverwertung und Fertilität adulter Gryllus bimaculatus. Oecologia **17** (1), 39–54, 1974.

Jacobs, W. und Renner, M. E.: Taschenlexikon zur Biologie der Insekten. Gustav Fischer Verlag, Stuttgart 1974.

Kaestner, A.: Lehrbuch der Speziellen Zoologie. Band I: Wirbellose, 1. Teil: Protozoa, Mesozoa, Parazoa, Coelenterata, Protostomia ohne Mandibulata. Gustav Fischer Verlag, Stuttgart 1965, 2. Aufl.

Kaestner, A.: Lehrbuch der Speziellen Zoologie. Band I: Wirbellose, 2. Teil: Crustacea. Gustav Fischer Verlag, Stuttgart 1967, 2. Aufl.

Kaltenbach, A.: Vorarbeiten für eine Revision der Phalangopsidae der äthiopischen Faunenregion (Saltatoria-Grylloidea). 3. Die zentralafrikanischen Arten der Gattung Phaeophilacris WALKER. Sber. Österr. Akad. Wiss., math.-naturw. KI., Abt. 1 **195**, 201–215, 1986.

Klcinsteuber, E.: Kleintiere im Terrarium. Wirbellose halten, züchten, kennenlernen. Urania-Verlag, Leipzig–Jena–Berlin 1989.

Löser, S.: Exotische Insekten, Tausendfüßer und Spinnentiere. Verlag Eugen Ulmer, Stuttgart 1991.

Martin, R. D., Rivers, J. P. and Cowgill, U. M.: Culturing mealworms as food for animals in captivity. Int. Zoo Yearbook **16,** 63–70, Dorchester 1976.

Mayer, H.: Zur Biologie und Ethologie einheimischer Collembolen. Zool. Jb., Syst. **85,** 501–570, 1957.

Mayer, M.: Kultur und Präparation der Protozoen. Franckh'sche Verlagshandlung, Stuttgart 1975, 5. Aufl.

Meinhardt, U.: Der unbekannte Regenwurm. Kosmos **78** (12), 48–54, 1982.

Menusan, H., Jr.: Effects of Temperature and Humidity on the Life Processes of the Bean Weevil, Bruchus obtectus SAY. Ann. ent. Soc. Amer. **27** (4), 515–526, 1934.

Menusan, H., Jr.: The Influence of Constant Temperatures and Humidities on the Rate of Growth and Relative Size of the Bean Weevil, Bruchus obtectus SAY. Ann. ent. Soc. Amer. **29** (2), 279–288, 1936.

Nutting, W. L.: Observations on the Reproduction of the Giant Cockroach, Blaberus craniifera BURM. Psyche **60,** 6–14, 1953.

Palissa, A.: Apterygota (Urinsekten). In: Brohmer, P., Ehrmann, P. und Ulmer, G.: leur. **4,** 1–407, Verlag Quelle & Meyer, Leipzig 1964.

Roth, I.. M.: Sexual Isolation in Parthenogenetic Pycnoscelus surinamensis and Application of the Name Pycnoscelus indicus to Its Bisexual Relative (Dictyoptera: aria: Blaberidae: Pycnoscelinae). Ann. ent. Soc. Amer. **60,** 774–779, 1967.

Roth, L. M. and Cohen, S. H.: Chromosomes of the Pycnoscelus indicus and P. surinamensis complex. (Blattaria: Blaberidae: Pycnoscelinae). Psyche **75** (1), 53–76, 1968.

Roth, L. M. and Willis, E. R.: Parthenogenesis in Cockroaches. Ann. ent. Soc. Amer. **49** (3), 195–204, 1956.

Roth, L. M. and Willis, E. R.: The Biology of Panchlora nivea, with Observations on the Eggs of Other Blattaria. Trans. Amer. ent. Soc. **83,** 195–207, 1958.

Roth, L. M. and Willis, E. R.: A Study of Bisexual and Parthenogenetic Strains of Pycnoscelus surinamensis (Blattaria: Epilamprinae). Ann. eiit. Soc. Amer.. **54**, 12–25, 1961.

Saupe, R.: Zur Kenntnis der Lebensweise der Riesenschabe Blabera fusca Brunner und der Gewächshausschabe Pycnoscelus surinamensis L. Z. angew. Ent. **14** (3), 461–500, 1929.

Schaller, F.: Collembola (Springschwänze). Handb. Zool. **4** (2) 2/1, 1–72, Verlag Walter de Gruyter, Berlin 1970.

Streble, H. und Krauter, D.: Das Leben im Wassertropfen. Franckh'sche Verlagshandlung, Stuttgart 1978, 4. Aufl.

Ude, H.: Oligochaeta, Hirudinea, Sipunculida. Tierw. Deutschl. **15**, 1–132, Verlag Gustav Fischer, Jena 1929.

Weidner, H.: Bestimmungstabellen der Vorratsschädlinge und des Hausungeziefers Mitteleuropas. Verlag Gustav Fischer, Jena 1937.

Wieser, W.: Die Bedeutung der Tageslänge für das Einsetzen der Fortpflanzungeperiode bei Porcellio scaber Latr [Isopoda]. Z. Naturfosch. **18b,** 1090–1092, 1963.

Willis, E. R., Riser, G. R. and Roth, L. M.: Observations on Reproduction and Development in Cockroaches. Ann. Ent. Soc. Amer. **51**, 53–69, 1958.

Zachariae, G.: Das Verhalten des Speisebohnenkäfers Acanthoscelides obtectus Say (Coleoptera: Bruchidae) im Freien in Norddeutschland. Z. angew. Ent. **43** (4). 345–365, 1958.

Zacher, F.: Untersuchungen zur Morphologie und Biologie der Samenkäfer (Bruchidae – Lariidae). Arb. a. d. Biol. Reichsanstalt Bd. **18,** H. 3, 233–384, 1930.

Zacher, F.: Verbreitung und Nährpflanzen des Speisebohnenkäfers, Acanthoscelides obtectus Say. Mitt. dt. ent. Ges. **14** (2), 3–4, 1955.

Zwart, P. and Rulkens, R. J.: Improving the calcium content of mealworms. Int. Zoo Yearbook **19**, 254–255, Dorchester 1979.

Image Sources

Drawings

Lindenbauer, Renate, Fig. 52
All other drawings by Klaus Ziegler †

Photographs

Lumpe, Hans: Figs. 23, 24, 27, 29, 30, 48, 49
Müller, Adolf: Fig. 18
All other photographs by Ursula Friedrich
The photographs in Fig. 4, 12, 32, 39, and 63 were taken at the Wilhelma Zoo in Stuttgart.

Index